CASE STUDIES
IN CLINICAL LABORATORY
SCIENCE

Linda Graves, Ed.D., M.T. (ASCP)

University of Maine at Presque Isle

With two contributors

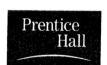

Prentice
Hall

Upper Saddle River, New Jersey 07458

Library of Congress Cataloging-in-Publication Data

Graves, Linda.
    Case studies in clinical laboratory science/Linda Graves.
        p. cm.
    Includes index.
    ISBN 0-13-088711-0
    1. Medical laboratory technology—Case studies.   I. Title.

RB37.5 .G73 2002
616.07'56—dc21   2001032109

Publisher: Julie Levin Alexander
CLS Series Editor: Elizabeth A. Zeibig
Senior Acquisitions Editor: Mark Cohen
Assistant Editor: Melissa Kerian
Marketing Manager: David Hough
Product Information Manager: Rachele Triano
**Director of Manufacturing
    and Production:** Bruce Johnson
Managing Production Editor: Patrick Walsh
Production Liaison: Mary Treacy

Production Editor: Janet Bolton
Manufacturing Manager: Ilene Sanford
Manufacturing Buyer: Pat Brown
Creative Director: Cheryl Asherman
Cover Design Coordinator: Maria Guglielmo Walsh
Interior Design/Composition: Janet Bolton
Electronic Art Creation: Electra Graphics
Printing and Binding: Courier Westford, Westford, MA
Proofreader: Maine Proofreading Services
Copy Editor: Louanne Elliott

Notice: The authors and the publisher of this textbook have taken care that the information and technical recommendations contained herein are based on research and expert consultation, and are accurate and compatible with the standards generally accepted at the time of publication. Nevertheless, as new information becomes available, changes in clinical and technical practices become necessary. The reader is advised to carefully consult manufacturers' instructions and information material for all supplies and equipment before use, and to consult with a health care professional as necessary. This advice is especially important when using new supplies or equipment for clinical purposes. The authors and publisher disclaim all responsibility for any liability, loss, injury, or damage incurred as a consequence, directly or indirectly, of the use and application of any of the contents of this volume.

Pearson Education LTD.
Pearson Education Australia PTY, Limited
Pearson Education Singapore, Pte. Ltd.
Pearson Education North Asia Ltd.
Pearson Education Canada, Ltd.
Pearson Educacion de Mexico, S.A. de C.V.
Pearson Education—Japan
Pearson Education Malaysia, Pte. Ltd.
Pearson Education, Upper Saddle River, New Jersey

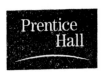

ISBN 0-13-088711-0

To my husband, Bill, who has encouraged and supported me throughout this project and understood when I was obsessed with deadlines. And to my students, who provided the initial impetus because of their love of case studies.

Contents

Preface

Case Studies in Clinical Laboratory Science was developed as a textbook to be used by students in the final semester or year of their 2- or 4-year clinical laboratory science programs. It will be most appropriate for students who have completed the didactic/theory portion of their education. Technicians and technologists who have been out of the field for awhile and are in the process of reentry into the profession, and technicians and technologists who are looking for a general review of clinical laboratory science will also find these cases a valuable exercise.

Case Studies in Clinical Laboratory Science consists of 55 cases in six main disciplines:

- 11 blood bank cases
- 12 chemistry cases
- 10 hematology cases
- 5 immunology cases
- 10 microbiology cases
- 7 urinalysis cases

Each case has

- A case presentation (including relevant data from the patient's medical history and physical examination as well as laboratory results)
- Questions
- References
- Answers

The answers are located in the appendix. Students will get more out of the exercise *if* they make a concerted effort to answer the questions *before* looking up the answers. If they are unable to answer the question from textbooks or class notes, the lists of references and suggested readings are sure to provide the relevant facts. Many of the references include Web sites that provide up-to-date information.

The cases provide an extensive review of important information in each of the areas. Many cases are multidisciplinary—tying together data from two, three, or four departments—to get students to see the big picture. Students often do not integrate the material from the various clinical laboratory disciplines as much as program directors and faculty would expect. Students don't make the connections between departments; each discipline remains in its own little box. These cases give students the opportunity to "experience" how departments work together to help the physician make a diagnosis and determine the best course of treatment for the patient. The cases are problem-solving and critical-thinking exercises, which also review pathophysiology (disease process), etiology (cause), and epidemiology. Questions like "What would you do next?" "What test(s) would the physician order?" "What other tests might be useful to determine the patient's status?" "Are these results consistent with other laboratory values or the patient's diagnosis?" give students the experience of making some of the decisions they will be making as laboratory professionals. They will be part of a health care team and should be ready to answer questions and provide physicians with the information they need.

These cases are also an excellent way for students to gain skills in researching and keeping up with the latest developments in clinical laboratory science. As we all know, the field is changing so fast that technicians and technologists who don't keep up with the latest developments are soon left behind. Clinical laboratory professionals need to be concerned with interpretation of data across disciplines, correlation of results to disease, problem solving, and quality assurance. *Case Studies in Clinical Laboratory Science* will provide readers with some experience dealing with "real" situations.

Foreword

The author and contributors of *Case Studies in Clinical Laboratory Science* present highly detailed and real-life case studies that will help learners envision themselves as members of the health care team—providing the laboratory aspects that assist in the patient care. These cases provide the opportunity to analyze and synthesize their technical skills. Learners are encouraged to use these cases not only to review their current knowledge but also to gain further insight into the exciting field of clinical laboratory science.

Case Studies in Clinical Laboratory Science is part of Prentice Hall's Clinical Laboratory Science series of textbooks, which is designed to balance theory and practical applications in a method that is engaging and useful to students. Furthermore, the books in this series are designed to foster various kinds of learning and some of the titles will be accompanied by computer applications.

We hope that this book, as well as the entire series, proves to be a valuable educational resource.

Elizabeth A. Zeibig
CLS Series Editor
Prentice Hall Health

FROM THE PUBLISHER

Prentice Hall would like to acknowledge the contributions of various educators who have served as focus group members over the past few years and who have assisted us in launching this series. We give special thanks to the following individuals:

Dianne M. Cearlock, Ph.D.
Professor and Director, Program in Clinical Laboratory Sciences
School of Allied Health Professions
Northern Illinois University
DeKalb, Illinois

Kathryn Doig, Ph.D., C.L.S. (NCA), C.L.S.p (H)
Program Director, Medical Technology Program
Michigan State University
East Lansing, Michigan

Linda Graves, Ed.D., M.T. (ASCP)
Program Director, Medical Laboratory Technology
University of Maine at Presque Isle
Presque Isle, Maine

Patricia K. Hargrave, Ph.D., C.L.S. (NCA), M.T. (ASCP)
Assistant Professor, Department of Clinical Laboratory Sciences
University of Kansas Medical Center
Kansas City, Kansas

Ellen M. Libby, M.S., M.T. (ASCP)
Program Director, Eastern Maine Medical Center
School of Medical Technology
Bangor, Maine

Harriet B. Mark, M.S., M.T. (ASCP)
Professor and Chair, Department of Clinical Laboratory Science
Associate Dean, College of Health Professions
SUNY Upstate Medical University
Syracuse, New York

Karen McClure, M.S., M.T. (ASCP)SBB
Director, Medical Technology Program
The University of Texas M.D. Anderson Cancer Center
Houston, Texas

Kay Paff, M.A., M.T. (ASCP)
Program Director, Medical Laboratory Technician
Kellogg Community College
Battle Creek, Michigan

Mary Jean Rutherford, M. Ed., M.T. (ASCP)SC
Program Director, Associate Professor
Clinical Laboratory Sciences Programs
Arkansas State University
State University, Arkansas

Teresa A. Taff, M.A., M.T. (ASCP)SM
Program Director, School of Clinical Laboratory Science
St. John's Mercy Medical Center
St. Louis, Missouri

Kathy V. Waller, Ph.D., C.L.S. (NCA)
Associate Professor, Medical Technology Division
The Ohio State University
Columbus, Ohio

Marcia A. Armstrong, M.S., M.T. (ASCP), C.L.S. (NCA)
Medical Laboratory Technician Program
Kapiolani Community College
Honolulu, Hawaii

Acknowledgments

I thank my contributors, Kathryn Doig and Frank Scarano, who were responsible for the hematology and microbiology chapters, respectively.

I also acknowledge the technologists who provided data for some of my case studies: Ellen LaChance, who provided the data and questions for four blood bank cases (1-5, 1-6, 1-7, and 1-10); Joan McElwain, who helped with information for three chemistry cases; and Jill Hatfield, who assisted with two blood bank cases.

Thank you to the technicians and technologists at my three clinical affiliates who keep me up-to-date on what's happening in the laboratory and interesting cases.

I thank my reviewers for their very helpful comments and suggestions: Larry S. Dunn, M.S., M.T. (ASCP), Program Director, Medical Laboratory Technology, Victoria College, Victoria, Texas; David Fowler, Ph.D., C.L.S. (NCA), Chair, Clinical Laboratory Sciences, University of Mississippi Medical Center, Jackson, Mississippi; Johanna W. Laird, M.S., M.T. (ASCP), Director, Clinical Laboratory Science/Medical Technology Program, Salisbury State University, Salisbury, Maryland; Jennifer Kellogg, M.T. (ASCP), Department of Medical Laboratory Technology, Arapahoe Community College, Littleton, Colorado; Ellen M. Libby, M.S., M.T. (ASCP), Program Director, Medical Technologist Program, Eastern Maine Medical Center, Bangor, Maine; Valerie Polansky, M.Ed., M.T. (ASCP), Program Director, Medical Laboratory Technology, St. Petersburg Junior College, St. Petersburg, Florida; and Venus Ward, Ph.D., M.T. (ASCP), Chair and Assistant Professor, Department of Clinical Laboratory Sciences, University of Kansas Medical Center, Kansas City, Kansas.

And last but not least, a special thanks to the editors and staff at Prentice-Hall. Mark Cohen, Acquisitions Editor, has been very supportive throughout this project. Beth Zeibig, Series Editor, provided helpful comments on various drafts and lots of support and encouragement. Her smiley faces on letters and reviews of case studies always made my day.

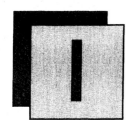

Blood Bank

BLOOD BANK CASE 1-1

Paul J., a 55-year-old man, was admitted with an intestinal obstruction. The following results were recorded by the blood bank technologist:

	Forward Grouping		Reverse Grouping		Rh Testing	
	Anti-A	Anti-B	A₁ Cells	B Cells	Anti-D	D Control
Paul J.	4+	1+	0	4+	3+	0

ANTIBODY SCREEN

	Screening Cell I				Screening Cell II				Screening Cell III				Autocontrol			
	IS	37	AHG	CC	IS	37	AHG	CC	IS	37	AHG	CC	IS	37	AHG	CC
Paul J.	0	0	0	4+	0	0	0	3+	0	0+	0	3+	0	0	0	4+

Abbreviations: IS, Immediate spin; 37, 37°C Incubation; AHG, Antihuman globulin; CC, Check cells.

QUESTIONS

1. What is Paul's probable ABO type?

2. What is the discrepant result in ABO grouping?

3. Explain the phenomenon that caused this pattern, and briefly describe two processes by which this can occur.

4. What bacteria are most commonly involved?

5. What steps would you take to confirm your suspicions?

6. Is the result of the antibody screen useful? Why or why not?

7.   a. Define secretor.

      b. What percent of the population are secretors?

c. Assuming he is SeSe, what ABO antigens will be present in Paul's secretions?

8. Will Paul's ABO reactions convert back to normal? If so, when?

RECOMMENDED READINGS

American Association of Blood Banks. (1999). *Technical Manual.* 13th ed. Bethesda, Md.: AABB.

Blaney, Kathy D. & Howard, Paula R. (2000). *Basic and Applied Concepts of Immunohematology.* St. Louis: Mosby.

Harmening, Denise M. (Ed.). (1999). *Modern Blood Banking and Transfusion Practices.* 4th ed. Philadelphia: F. A. Davis.

Quinley, Eva D. (1998). *Immunohematology: Principles and Practice.* 2nd ed. Philadelphia: J. B. Lippincott.

BLOOD BANK CASE I–2

Lisa N., a 25-year-old woman pregnant with her second child, had routine orders for a "type and screen," with the following results:

	Forward Grouping		Reverse Grouping		Rh Testing	
	Anti-A	Anti-B	A Cells	B Cells	Anti-D	D Control
Lisa N.	3+	0	0	4+	4+	0

ANTIBODY SCREEN

	Screening Cell I				Screening Cell II				Screening Cell III				Autocontrol			
	IS	37	AHG	CC	IS	37	AHG	CC	IS	37	AHG	CC	IS	37	AHG	CC
Lisa N.	0	0	0	4+	0	2+	3+		0	2+	3+		0	0	0	4+

Abbreviations: IS, Immediate spin; 37, 37°C Incubation; AHG, Antihuman globulin; CC, Check cells.

QUESTIONS

1. What is Lisa's blood type?

2. What would be the interpretation of the antibody screen?

3. What immunoglobulin class is the most probable for this antibody?

4. Is the antibody an alloantibody and/or autoantibody? Can either be ruled out? Explain.

5. What detail in the patient history would provide further evidence for your answer to question 4?

6. What procedure would the technologist perform next?

7. How are antibodies ruled out in the cross-out method of antibody panel interpretation? Explain the procedure in two or three sentences.

Review Figure 1–1, "Antibody Panel, Case 1–2." In this case study, antibodies are excluded only if the patient's serum does not react with panel cells that are *homozygous* for the antigen.

8. Why are antibodies ruled out only when there is no reaction with homozygous cells?

Figure 1–1.   ANTIBODY PANEL, CASE 1–2

No.	Rh	Rhesus								MNS				P	Lewis		Lutheran		Kell				Duffy		Kidd			LISS			
		D	C	E	c	e	f	Cw	V	M	N	S	s	P1	Lea	Leb	Lua	Lub	K	k	Kpa	Jsa	Fya	Fyb	Jka	Jkb	Xga	IS	37	AHG	CC
1	rr	0	0	0	+	+	+	0	0	0	+	+	+	+	+	0	0	+	0	+	0	0	0	+	0	+	+	0	2+	3+	
2	rr	0	0	0	+	+	+	0	0	+	0	0	+	+	0	+	0	+	+	+	0	0	0	+	+	0	0	0	2+	3+	
3	r'r	0	+	0	+	+	+	0	0	0	+	0	+	+s	0	+	0	+	0	+	0	+	+	0	+	0	0	0	2+	3+	
4	r''r	0	0	+	+	+	+	0	0	0	+	+	0	+	0	+	0	+	0	+	0	0	+	+	+	0	0	0	2+	3+	
5	rr	0	0	0	+	+	+	0	0	+	0	+	+	+	0	0	0	+	0	+	0	0	+	+	+	+	+	0	2+	3+	
6	R0r	+	0	0	+	+	+	0	+	+	0	0	+	+s	0	0	0	+	0	+	0	0	0	0	+	0	+	0	2+	3+	
7	R1R1	+	+	0	0	+	NT	0	0	+	+	0	+	0	+	0	0	+	+	+	+	0	+	+	0	+	0	0	0	0	3+
8	R1R1	+	+	0	0	+	NT	0	0	+	+	+	0	+w	0	+	0	+	+	+	0	0	0	+	+	+	0	0	0	0	3+
9	R1R1	+	+	0	0	+	NT	+	0	+	+	0	+	+s	0	+	0	+	0	+	0	0	0	+	+	0	+	0	0	0	3+
10	R2R2	+	0	+	+	0	NT	0	0	0	0	0	+	+vs	0	+	0	+	0	0	0	0	0	+	0	+	+	0	2+	3+	
11	R1r	+	+	0	+	+	+	0	0	+	0	+	+	0	0	+	+	0	0	0	0	+	0	+	+	+	+	0	2+	3+	
AC																												0	0	0	4+

No.	Rh	Rhesus								MNS				P	Lewis		Lutheran		Kell				Duffy		Kidd			LISS			
		D	C	E	c	e	f	Cw	V	M	N	S	s	P1	Lea	Leb	Lua	Lub	K	k	Kpa	Jsa	Fya	Fyb	Jka	Jkb	Xga	IS	37	AHG	CC
SCI		+	+	0	0	+	0	+	0	+	+	+	0	+	0	+	0	+	+	+	0	0	+	+	+	0	+	0	0	0	4+
SCII		+	0	+	+	0	0	0	0	0	0	0	+	+	+	0	0	+	0	+	0	+	+	0	+	+	+	0	2+	3+	
SCIII		0	0	0	+	+	+	0	0	0	+	0	+	+	+	0	0	+	0	+	0	0	0	0	0	+	+	0	2+	3+	

vs: very strong
s: strong
NT: not tested
AC: autocontrol
vw: very weak
w: weak

LISS: Low-ionic Strength Saline
SCI: Screening Cell I
SCII: Screening Cell II
SCIII: Screening Cell III

9. What antibody(ies) cannot be ruled out by the panel results?

10. What is/are the most likely antibody(ies)? Why?

11.   a. Discuss the 3 + 3 Rule (Rule of Three).

      b. Do(es) the antibodies(y) you identified in Question 10 meet the 3 + 3 Rule?

Lisa N. was phenotyped for the following antigens:

	Anti-C	Anti-c	Anti-E	Anti-e	Anti-K
Lisa N.	3+	0	2+	2+	3+

12.   a. What is Lisa's Fisher-Race phenotype?

b. Does Lisa's antigen phenotype confirm or conflict with your antibody identification?

13. Does the screening cell antigram (see Figure 1–1) confirm or refute your antibody identification?

14. How would you rule out the remaining antibodies?

15. If Lisa required crossmatching for 3 U, what additional step would be added to the crossmatch procedure?

RECOMMENDED READINGS

American Association of Blood Banks. (1999). *Technical Manual.* 13th ed. Bethesda, Md.: AABB.

Blaney, Kathy D. & Howard, Paula R. (2000). *Basic and Applied Concepts of Immunohematology.* St. Louis: Mosby.

Harmening, Denise M. (Ed.). (1999). *Modern Blood Banking and Transfusion Practices.* 4th ed. Philadelphia: F. A. Davis.

Quinley, Eva D. (1998). *Immunohematology: Principles and Practice.* 2nd ed. Philadelphia: J. B. Lippincott.

BLOOD BANK CASE 1–3

Jim S., a 55-year-old man, was admitted to the hospital for cardiac bypass surgery. His physician ordered a type and crossmatch for 5 U. The blood bank technologist recorded the following results:

	Forward Grouping		Reverse Grouping		Rh Testing	
	Anti-A	Anti-B	A Cells	B Cells	Anti-D	D Control
Jim S.	0	0	4+	4+	3+	0

ANTIBODY SCREEN

	Screening Cell I				Screening Cell II				Screening Cell III				Autocontrol			
	IS	37	AHG	CC	IS	37	AHG	CC	IS	37	AHG	CC	IS	37	AHG	CC
Jim S.	0	1+	4+		0	2+	3+		0	0	0	3+	0	0	0	4+

Abbreviations: IS, Immediate spin; 37, 37°C Incubation; AHG, Antihuman globulin; CC, Check cells.

QUESTIONS

1. What is Jim's blood type?

2. What is your interpretation of the antibody screen?

3. What immunoglobulin class is/are the antibody(ies)? Explain.

Review Figure 1–2, "Antibody Panel, Case 1–3." In this case study, antibodies are excluded only if the patient's serum does not react with panel cells that are *homozygous* for the antigen.

4. What antibody(ies) cannot be ruled out by the panel results?

5. Is any antibody in question 3 a perfect match for the panel results?

6. What are some possible explanations for the panel results?

7. What is the *most likely* explanation for the panel results?

Figure 1–2.   ANTIBODY PANEL, CASE 1–3

No.	Rh	Rhesus D	C	E	c	e	f	Cw	V	MNS M	N	S	s	P P1	Lewis Lea	Leb	Lutheran Lua	Lub	Kell K	k	Kpa	Jsa	Duffy Fya	Fyb	Kidd Jka	Jkb	Xga	LISS IS	37	AHG	CC
1	rr	0	0	0	+	+	+	0	0	0	+	0	+	+	+	0	0	+	0	+	0	0	0	+	+	0	+	0	0	0	3+
2	rr	0	0	0	+	+	+	0	0	+	+	0	+	+	+	0	0	+	+	+	0	0	0	+	0	+	0	0	3+	4+	
3	r'r	0	+	0	+	+	+	0	0	+	0	+	+	+s	+	0	0	+	0	+	0	0	+	0	+	+	+	0	0	0	3+
4	r''r	0	0	+	+	+	+	0	0	+	+	0	+	+	0	+	+	+	0	+	0	0	+	+	0	+	+	0	1+	3+	
5	rr	0	0	0	+	+	+	0	0	+	0	0	0	0	0	+	0	+	0	+	0	0	+	+	+	+	+	0	0	0	3+
6	R0r	+	0	0	+	+	+	0	+	+	0	0	+	+s	0	0	0	+	0	+	0	0	0	0	+	0	+	0	0	0	3+
7	R1R1	+	+	0	0	+	NT	0	0	+	+	0	+	0	0	+	0	+	0	+	0	0	0	+	0	0	+	0	0	0	3+
8	R1R1	+	+	0	0	+	0	0	0	0	+	0	+	+w	0	+	0	+	0	+	0	0	+	0	+	0	+	0	3+	4+	
9	R1R1	+	+	0	0	+	NT	+	0	+	+	+	+	+s	+	0	0	+	+	+	0	0	+	0	+	+	+	0	0	0	3+
10	R2R2	+	0	+	+	0	NT	0	0	0	+	0	+	+vs	0	+	0	+	0	+	0	0	0	+	0	+	+	0	1+	3+	
11	R1r	+	+	0	+	+	+	0	0	+	+	+	+	+	+	0	+	+	+	+	0	0	+	+	+	+	+	0	3+	4+	
AC		+	+	0	+	+														0								0	0	0	3+

No.	Rh	Rhesus D	C	E	c	e	f	Cw	V	MNS M	N	S	s	P P1	Lewis Lea	Leb	Lutheran Lua	Lub	Kell K	k	Kpa	Jsa	Duffy Fya	Fyb	Kidd Jka	Jkb	Xga	IS	37	AHG	CC
SCI		+	+	0	0	+	0	+	0	+	+	+	0	+	0	+	0	+	+	+	0	0	0	+	+	+	0	0	1+	4+	
SCII		+	0	+	+	0	0	0	0	+	0	0	+	+	+	0	0	+	0	+	0	+	+	0	+	+	+	0	2+	3+	
SCIII		0	0	0	+	+	+	0	+	0	+	0	+	+	+	0	0	+	0	+	0	0	+	0	0	+	+	0	0	0	3+

vs: very strong
s: strong
NT: not tested
AC: autocontrol
vw: very weak
w: weak

8. What is/are the most likely antibody(ies)?

9. What three confirmatory procedures are used to confirm antibody identification?

10. Do any of the confirmatory procedures in question 9 (that are available to
    you) confirm or rule out the antibody or antibodies in question 8?

11. How would you rule out the remaining antibodies?

12. Explain how the technologist would proceed to find compatible units for crossmatch.

13.   a. Approximately what percentage of units would be compatible?

   b. How many units would have to be phenotyped to find 5 compatible units?

RECOMMENDED READINGS

American Association of Blood Banks. (1999). *Technical Manual*. 13th ed. Bethesda, Md.: AABB.

Blaney, Kathy D. & Howard, Paula R. (2000). *Basic and Applied Concepts of Immunohematology*. St. Louis: Mosby.

Harmening, Denise M. (Ed.). (1999). *Modern Blood Banking and Transfusion Practices*. 4th ed. Philadelphia: F. A. Davis.

Quinley, Eva D. (1998). *Immunohematology: Principles and Practice*. 2nd ed. Philadelphia: J. B. Lippincott.

BLOOD BANK CASE 1–4

Ruth N., a 90-year-old woman, required a crossmatch for 4 U. The blood bank technologist recorded the following results:

	Forward Type		Re verse Type		Rh Typing	
	Anti-A	Anti-B	A Cells	B Cells	Anti-D	D Control
Ruth N.	3+	0	0	2+	3+	0

ANTIBODY SCREEN

	Screening Cell I				Screening Cell II				Screening Cell III				Autocontrol			
	IS	37	AHG	CC	IS	37	AHG	CC	IS	37	AHG	CC	IS	37	AHG	CC
Ruth N.	0	0	3+		0	0	±		0	0	2+		0	0	0	2+

Abbreviations: IS, Immediate spin; 37, 37°C Incubation; AHG, Antihuman globulin; CC, Check cells.

QUESTIONS

1. What is Ruth's blood type?

2. What is the result (interpretation) of the antibody screen?

3. Does Ruth have an alloantibody(ies) and/or autoantibody(ies)? Explain your answer.

Review Figure 1–3. In this case study, antibodies are excluded only if the patient's serum does not react with panel cells that are *homozygous* for the antigen.

Figure 1-3. ANTIBODY PANEL, CASE 1-4, PERFORMED BY TUBE METHOD

No.	Rh	Rhesus								Kell						Duffy		Kidd		Sex Linked	Lewis		MNS				P	Lutheran		LISS			
		D	C	E	c	e	f	C^w	V	K	k	Kp^a	Kp^b	Js^a	Js^b	Fy^a	Fy^b	Jk^a	Jk^b	Xg^a	Le^a	Le^b	S	s	M	N	P$_1$	Lu^a	Lu^b	IS	37	AHG	CC
1	rr	0	0	0	+	+	+	0	0	+	+	+	0	0	+	0	+	0	+	+	0	+	0	+	+	+	0	0	+	0	0	3+	
2	rr	0	0	0	+	+	+	0	0	0	+	0	+	0	+	+	0	+	0	+	0	+	0	+	+	+	+	0	+	0	0	+/−	
3	rr	0	0	0	+	+	+	0	0	0	+	+	0	0	+	0	+	0	+	+	+	0	+	+	+	+	+	0	+	0	0	0	2+
4	R$_2$R$_2$	+	0	+	0	0	0	0	0	0	+	0	+	0	+	+	0	+	+	+	0	+	+	+	0	+	+	0	+	0	0	+/−	
5	R$_2$R$_2$	+	0	+	0	0	0	0	0	0	+	0	+	0	+	0	+	+	0	+	0	+	+	+	0	+	+	0	+	0	0	1+	
6	R$_2$R$_2$	+	0	+	0	0	0	0	0	+	+	0	+	0	+	+	+	0	+	+	+	0	0	+	+	+	+	0	+	0	0	0	2+
7	R$_1$R$_1$	+	+	0	0	+	0	0	0	0	+	+	0	0	+	+	0	+	+	+	+	0	+	0	+	0	+	0	+	0	0	0	2+
8	R$_1$R$_1$	+	+	0	0	+	0	0	0	+	+	0	+	+	0	0	+	0	+	+	0	+	0	+	0	+	+	0	+	0	0	?0	2+
9	R$_2$R$_1$	+	+	+	0	+	+	0	0	+	+	0	+	0	+	0	+	+	0	+	0	+	+	+	+	0	+	0	+	0	0	2+	
10	r'r	0	+	0	+	+	+	0	0	0	+	0	+	0	+	+	+	+	+	+	0	+	0	0	+	0	+	0	+	0	0	+/−	
11	R$_1$R$_1$	+	+	0	0	+	0	0	0	+	0	0	+	0	+	+	+	0	+	+	0	+	+	+	+	+	+	0	+	0	0	3+	
AC		0	0	0	0	0	0	0	0	0	0	0	+	+	0	+	+	0	0	0	0	0								0	0	0	2+

No.	Rh	Rhesus								Kell						Duffy		Kidd		Sex Linked	Lewis		MNS				P	Lutheran		LISS			
		D	C	E	c	e	f	C^w	V	K	k	Kp^a	Kp^b	Js^a	Js^b	Fy^a	Fy^b	Jk^a	Jk^b	Xg^a	Le^a	Le^b	S	s	M	N	P$_1$	Lu^a	Lu^b	IS	37	AHG	CC
SCI	R$_1$R$_1$	+	+	0	0	+	0	0	0	+	+	+	+	0	+	0	+	+	0	+	0	+	0	+	+	0	0	0	+	0	0	3+	
SCII	R$_2$R$_2$	+	0	+	+	0	0	0	0	0	+	+	0	0	+	+	0	+	+	+	0	+	+	+	+	+	+	0	+	0	0	+/−	
SCIII	rr	0	0	0	0	+	+	+	0	0	0	+	0	+	0	+	+	0	0	+	0	+	+	0	+	0	0	0	+	0	0	0	2+

4. What antibodies cannot be ruled out in Figure 1–3 using the conventional tube method? (Do *not* use cell 8 as a rule-out cell, because the technologist had a question.)

Review the screening cell antigram in Figure 1–3.

5. What antibodies cannot be ruled out with the screening cell antigram?

6. Does the screening cell antigram rule out any antibodies that are not eliminated by the panel in Figure 1–3?

Review Figure 1–4.

7. What antibodies cannot be ruled out in Figure 1–4 using the gel method?

Figure I–4.   ANTIBODY PANEL, CASE I–4, PERFORMED BY GEL METHOD

No.	Rh	Rhesus								Kell						Duffy		Kidd		Sex Linked	Lewis		MNS				P	Lutheran		IS	37	AHG	CC
		D	C	E	c	e	f	C^w	V	K	k	Kp^a	Kp^b	Js^a	Js^b	Fy^a	Fy^b	Jk^a	Jk^b	Xg^a	Le^a	Le^b	S	s	M	N	P_1	Lu^a	Lu^b	IS	37	AHG	CC
1	R_1R_1	+	+	0	0	+	0	+	0	0	+	0	+	0	+	+	0	+	0	+	0	+	0	+	0	+	+	0	+	0	0	1+	
2	R_1R_1	+	+	0	0	+	0	0	0	+	+	0	+	0	+	+	0	0	+	+	0	0	0	+	0	+	0	0	+	0	0	2+	
3	R_2R_2	+	0	+	+	0	0	0	0	0	+	0	+	0	+	0	+	+	+	+	+	0	0	+	+	+	+	0	+	0	0	+/–	
4	R_0r	+	0	0	+	+	+	0	+	0	+	0	+	0	+	0	0	+	0	+	0	0	+	+	+	0	+	0	+	0	0	+/–	
5	r'r	0	+	0	+	+	+	0	0	0	+	0	+	0	+	0	+	0	+	+	+	0	+	+	+	0	+	0	+	0	0	0	2+
6	r''r	0	0	+	+	+	+	0	0	+	+	0	+	0	+	+	+	+	+	+	0	+	0	+	+	0	0	0	+	0	0	3+	
7	rr	0	0	0	+	+	+	0	0	+	+	0	+	0	+	0	+	+	+	+	0	+	+	+	+	0	+	0	+	0	0	2+	2+
8	rr	0	0	0	+	+	+	0	0	0	+	0	+	0	+	+	+	0	+	+	0	+	+	0	+	0	+	0	+	0	0	0	2+
9	rr	0	0	0	+	+	+	0	0	0	+	0	+	0	+	+	0	+	0	+	+	0	0	+	+	+	0	0	+	0	0	1+	
10	rr	0	0	0	+	+	+	0	0	0	+	0	+	0	+	+	0	+	0	0	0	0	0	+	0	+	+	0	+	0	0	1+	
11	R_1R_1	+	+	0	0	+	0	0	0	0	+	0	+	0	+	+	+	+	+	0	0	+	+	0	+	+	+	0	+	0	0	0	2+
AC																														0	0	0	2+

No.	Rh	Rhesus								Kell						Duffy		Kidd		Sex Linked	Lewis		MNS				P	Lutheran		IS	37	AHG	CC
		D	C	E	c	e	f	C^w	V	K	k	Kp^a	Kp^b	Js^a	Js^b	Fy^a	Fy^b	Jk^a	Jk^b	Xg^a	Le^a	Le^b	S	s	M	N	P_1	Lu^a	Lu^b	IS	37	AHG	CC
SCI	R_1R_1	+	+	0	0	+	0	0	0	+	+	+	+	0	+	0	+	+	0	+	0	+	0	+	+	0	0	0	+	0			
SCII	R_2R_2	+	0	+	+	0	0	0	0	0	+	0	+	0	+	+	0	+	+	+	0	+	+	+	+	+	+	0	+	0			
SCIII	rr	0	0	0	+	+	+	+	0	0	0	+	0	+	0	+	+	+	0	+	0	+	+	0	+	0	0	0	+	0			

8. If the results of Figures 1–3 and 1–4 and the antibody screen are combined, what antibodies cannot be ruled out?

9. What are the most likely antibodies (two or more antibodies that match the panel reactions perfectly)?

10. Does the following antigen typing confirm or refute your answer?

	Anti-K	Anti-Fyᵃ	Anti-Jkᵃ
Ruth N.	0	2+	0

RECOMMENDED READINGS

American Association of Blood Banks. (1999). *Technical Manual*. 13th ed. Bethesda, Md.: AABB.

Blaney, Kathy D. & Howard, Paula R. (2000). *Basic and Applied Concepts of Immunohematology*. St. Louis: Mosby.

Harmening, Denise M. (Ed.). (1999). *Modern Blood Banking and Transfusion Practices*. 4th ed. Philadelphia: F. A. Davis.

Quinley, Eva D. (1998). *Immunohematology: Principles and Practice*. 2nd ed. Philadelphia: J. B. Lippincott.

BLOOD BANK CASE 1–5*

A physician ordered a type and crossmatch for 3 U on Mary G., a 50-year-old woman who was scheduled for elective surgery.

The blood bank technologist recorded the following results:

	Forward Grouping		Reverse Grouping		Rh Testing	
	Anti-A	Anti-B	A Cells	B Cells	Anti-D	D Control
Mary G.	3+	0	0	2+	3+	0

QUESTIONS

1. What are Mary's ABO and Rh?

Review the antibody screen results on the bottom of Figure 1–5.

2. Does Mary have an alloantibody(ies) and/or autoantibody(ies)? Explain your answer.

3. What antibodies cannot be ruled out with the screening cell antigram?

Review Figure 1–5. In this case study, antibodies are excluded only if the patient's serum does not react with panel cells that are *homozygous* for the antigen.

* Data and sample questions courtesy of Ellen O. LaChance, M.S., M.T. (ASCP), S.B.B., Supervisor of Transfusion Service, Affiliated Laboratory/Eastern Maine Medical Center, Bangor, Maine.

Figure I–5. ANTIBODY PANEL, CASE I–5, PERFORMED BY TUBE METHOD

No.	Rh	Rhesus								Kell						Duffy		Kidd		Sex Linked	Lewis		MNS				P	Lutheran		LISS			
		D	C	E	c	e	f	C^W	V	K	k	Kp^a	Kp^b	Js^a	Js^b	Fy^a	Fy^b	Jk^a	Jk^b	Xg^a	Le^a	Le^b	S	s	M	N	P_1	Lu^a	Lu^b	IS	37	AHG	CC
1	R_1R_1	+	+	0	0	+	0	+	0	0	+	0	+	0	+	+	+	0	+	+	+	0	0	+	+	+	+	0	+	0	0	2+	
2	R_1R_1	+	+	0	0	+	0	0	0	+	+	0	+	0	+	+	+	0	+	+	0	+	+	+	+	+	+	0	+	0	0	3+	
3	R_2R_2	+	0	+	+	0	0	0	0	0	+	0	+	0	+	+	0	+	+	+	0	+	0	+	0	+	+	0	+	0	0	2+	
4	R_0r	+	0	0	+	+	+	0	+	0	+	0	+	0	+	0	0	+	0	+	0	0	0	+	+	0	+	0	+	0	0	0	2+
5	r'r	0	+	0	+	+	+	0	0	0	+	0	+	0	+	+	+	+	0	0	0	+	+	0	+	0	0	0	+	0	0	3+	
6	r''r	0	0	+	+	+	+	0	0	+	+	0	+	0	+	0	+	0	+	+	0	+	+	+	+	+	+	0	+	0	0	2+	
7	rr	0	0	0	+	+	+	0	0	+	+	0	+	0	+	0	+	+	+	+	0	0	0	+	+	+	0	0	+	0	0	2+	
8	rr	0	0	0	+	+	+	0	0	0	+	0	+	0	+	+	+	+	+	0	+	0	+	+	+	0	+	0	+	0	0	3+	
9	rr	0	0	0	+	+	+	0	0	0	+	0	+	0	+	+	+	+	0	+	0	+	0	+	0	+	+	0	+	0	0	3+	
10	rr	0	0	0	+	+	+	0	0	0	+	0	+	0	+	0	+	+	0	+	0	0	+	0	+	+	+	0	+	0	0	0	2+
11	R_1R_1	+	+	0	0	0	0	0	0	0	+	0	+	0	+	0	+	+	0	0	0	0	+	+	+	0	+	0	+	0	0	0	2+
AC																														0	0	0	3+

No.	Rh	Rhesus								Kell						Duffy		Kidd		Sex Linked	Lewis		MNS				P	Lutheran		LISS			
		D	C	E	c	e	f	C^W	V	K	k	Kp^a	Kp^b	Js^a	Js^b	Fy^a	Fy^b	Jk^a	Jk^b	Xg^a	Le^a	Le^b	S	s	M	N	P_1	Lu^a	Lu^b	IS	37	AHG	CC
SCI	R_1R_1	+	+	0	0	+	0	0	0	0	+	0	+	0	+	+	0	0	+	+	+	0	0	+	+	0	+	0	+	0	0	2+	
SCII	R_2R_2	+	0	+	+	0	0	0	0	0	+	0	+	0	+	0	+	+	0	0	0	+	+	+	0	+	+	0	+	0	0	0	2+
SCIII	rr	0	0	0	+	+	+	0	0	+	+	0	+	0	+	+	0	+	+	+	0	+	+	+	+	+	0	0	+	0	0	3+	

AC: autocontrol

4. What antibodies cannot be ruled out with the antibody panel in Figure 1–5?

5. What antibodies cannot be ruled out by either the antibody screen or antibody panel in Figure 1–5?

6. What antigens are enhanced by the addition of ficin or papain? What antigens are inactivated?

7. Discuss the effect of polyethylene glycol (PEG) on the antihuman globulin procedure?

Review the antibody panel in Figure 1–6 (ImmuAdd + ficin, PEG).

8. What antibody(ies) is/are identified by the enzyme-treated (ImmuAdd ficin AHG, PEG) panel (Figure 1–6)? What antibodies cannot be ruled out?

Figure 1–6.   ANTIBODY PANEL, CASE 1–5, PERFORMED BY GEL METHOD

No.	Rh	Rhesus								Kell						Duffy		Kidd		Sex Linked	Lewis		MNS				P	Lutheran		ImmuAdd ficin AHG		ImmuAdd + AHG, PEG		ImmuAdd AHG + PEG	
		D	C	E	c	e	f	C^w	V	K	k	Kp^a	Kp^b	Js^a	Js^b	Fy^a	Fy^b	Jk^a	Jk^b	Xg^a	Le^a	Le^b	S	s	M	N	P_1	Lu^a	Lu^b	AHG	CC	AHG	CC	AHG	CC
1	R_1R_1	+	+	0	0	+	0	+	0	0	+	0	+	0	+	+	+	0	+	+	+	0	0	+	+	+	+	0	+	0	2+	0	2+	3+	
2	R_1R_1	+	+	0	0	+	0	0	0	+	+	0	+	0	+	+	+	0	+	+	0	+	+	+	+	+	+	0	+	3+		3+		3+	
3	R_2R_2	+	0	+	+	0	0	0	0	0	+	0	+	0	+	+	0	+	+	+	0	+	0	+	0	0	+	0	+	0	2+	0	2+	2+	
4	R_0r	+	0	0	+	+	+	0	+	0	+	0	+	0	+	0	0	+	0	+	0	0	0	+	+	0	+	0	+	0	2+	0	2+	0	2+
5	r'r	0	+	0	+	+	+	0	0	0	+	0	+	0	+	+	+	+	0	0	0	+	+	0	+	0	0	0	+	0	2+	0	2+	3+	
6	r"r	0	0	+	+	+	+	0	0	+	+	0	+	0	+	0	+	0	+	+	0	+	+	+	+	+	+	0	+	2+		2+		2+	
7	rr	0	0	0	+	+	+	0	0	0	+	0	+	0	+	0	0	+	+	+	+	+	0	+	+	+	0	0	+	2+		2+		2+	
8	rr	0	0	0	+	+	+	0	0	0	+	0	+	0	+	+	+	+	+	0	0	+	0	+	0	0	+	0	+	0	2+	0	2+	2+	
9	rr	0	0	0	+	+	+	0	0	0	+	0	+	0	+	+	0	0	0	+	0	0	0	+	+	+	+	0	+	0	2+	0	2+	0	2+
10	rr	0	0	0	+	+	+	0	0	0	+	0	+	0	+	0	+	+	+	+	0	0	+	0	+	+	+	0	+	0	2+	0	2+	0	2+
11	R_1R_1	+	+	0	0	+	0	0	0	0	+	0	+	0	+	0	+	+	0	0	0	+	+	+	+	0	+	0	+	0	2+	0	2+	0	2+

9. Using a different color pen/pencil from the one you used in question 8 (so you can tell what antibodies are ruled out by this panel), what antibody(ies) is/are identified by the ImmuAdd AHG PEG panel (Figure 1–6)? What antibodies cannot be ruled out?

The following antigen typing was performed on Mary's red blood cells (RBCs):

	Rh					Kell	Duffy	
	Anti-D	Anti-C	Anti-E	Anti-c	Anti-e	Anti-K	Anti-Fy^a	Anti-Fy^b
Mary G.	4+	0	3+	3+	0	0	0	3+

10. What is Mary's most probable Rh genotype?

11. Do the antigen typing results support or rule out your panel results—the most probable antibody(ies)?

12. How many units should the technologist type to find 3 compatible units?

RECOMMENDED READINGS

American Association of Blood Banks. (1999). *Technical Manual.* 13th ed. Bethesda, Md.: AABB.

Blaney, Kathy D. & Howard, Paula R. (2000). *Basic and Applied Concepts of Immunohematology.* St. Louis: Mosby.

Harmening, Denise M. (Ed.). (1999). *Modern Blood Banking and Transfusion Practices.* 4th ed. Philadelphia: F. A. Davis.

Quinley, Eva D. (1998). *Immunohematology: Principles and Practice.* 2nd ed. Philadelphia: J. B. Lippincott.

BLOOD BANK CASE 1–6*

Jane S. was admitted for a redo of a hip arthroplasty and had an order for 2 U of packed RBCs. She received 2 U of packed RBCs 1 year prior when she had the original hip surgery. Jane typed as A positive, and a review of her transfusion history found no prior history of alloantibodies. She was transfused with 1 U of packed RBCs during surgery.

Review Figure 1–7, antibody screen 1, done on 11/21/00.

QUESTIONS

1. Does the antibody screen indicate the presence of any alloantibodies?

On 11/28/00, a type and crossmatch were ordered because the patient's hemoglobin and hematocrit were dropping.

Preop hemoglobin and hematocrit	11.9 g/dL (reference range, 12 to 16 g/dL); 35.6% (reference range, 37 to 47%)
11/28/00 hemoglobin and hematocrit	8.0 g/dL; 24.1%

2. What is the most likely explanation for the drop in hemoglobin and hematocrit?

Review Figure 1–7, antibody screen 2, done on 11/28/00.

3. Does the postoperative antibody screen indicate the presence of any alloantibodies?

---

* Data and sample questions courtesy of Ellen O. LaChance, M.S., M.T. (ASCP), S.B.B., Supervisor of Transfusion Service, Affiliated Laboratory/Eastern Maine Medical Center, Bangor, Maine.

Figure 1-7. ANTIBODY SCREENS, CASE 1-6

Antibody Screen 1   11/21/00

No.	Rh	Rhesus								Kell						Duffy		Kidd		Sex Linked	Lewis		MNS				P	Lutheran		37	AHG	CC
		D	C	E	c	e	f	C^w	V	K	k	Kp^a	Kp^b	Js^a	Js^b	Fy^a	Fy^b	Jk^a	Jk^b	Xg^a	Le^a	Le^b	S	s	M	N	P$_1$	Lu^a	Lu^b	37	AHG	CC
SCI	R$_1$R$_1$	+	+	0	0	+	0	0	0	+	+	0	+	0	+	+	0	+	+	0	0	+	0	+	+	+	+	0	+	0	0	3+
SCII	R$_2$R$_2$	+	0	+	+	0	0	0	0	0	+	0	+	0	+	+	+	+	0	+	+	0	+	+	0	+	+	0	+	0	0	3+
AC																														0	0	3+

Antibody Screen 2   11/28/00

No.	Rh	Rhesus								Kell						Duffy		Kidd		Sex Linked	Lewis		MNS				P	Lutheran		37	AHG	CC
		D	C	E	c	e	f	C^w	V	K	k	Kp^a	Kp^b	Js^a	Js^b	Fy^a	Fy^b	Jk^a	Jk^b	Xg^a	Le^a	Le^b	S	s	M	N	P$_1$	Lu^a	Lu^b	37	AHG	CC
SCI	R$_1$R$_1$	+	+	0	0	+	0	0	0	+	+	0	+	0	+	+	0	+	+	0	0	+	0	+	+	+	+	0	+	0	2+	
SCII	R$_2$R$_2$	+	0	+	+	0	0	0	0	0	+	0	+	0	+	+	+	+	0	+	+	0	+	+	0	+	+	0	+	0	0	2+
AC																														0	1+	

NT: not tested
AC: autocontrol

4. What is the significance of the positive autocontrol?

A direct antiglobulin panel was performed because of the positive auto-control.

	IS	5'	CC
Polyspecific AHG	1+	1+	
Anti-IgG	1+	1+	
Anti-C3	0	0	3+

5. a. Explain the results of the direct antiglobulin panel.

b. What would you do next?

Review Figure 1–8, "Antibody Panel, Case 1–6." In this case study, antibodies are excluded only if the patient's serum does not react with panel cells that are *homozygous* for the antigen.

6. What antibodies cannot be ruled out by the antibody panel in Figure 1–8?

Figure 1–8. ANTIBODY PANEL, CASE 1–6

No.	Rh	D	C	E	c	e	f	Cw	V	K	k	Kpa	Kpb	Jsa	Jsb	Fya	Fyb	Jka	Jkb	Xga	Lea	Leb	S	s	M	N	P1	Lua	Lub	37	AHG	CC	Elution
		Rhesus								**Kell**						**Duffy**		**Kidd**		**Sex Linked**	**Lewis**		**MNS**				**P**	**Lutheran**		**LISS**			
1	R1R1	+	+	0	0	+	0	+	0	0	+	0	+	0	+	0	+	0	+	+	0	+	+	+	+	+	+	0	+	0	3+		1+
2	R1R1	+	+	0	0	+	0	0	0	+	+	0	+	0	+	+	+	0	+	+	+	0	0	+	+	0	+	0	+	0	3+		1+
3	R2R2	+	0	+	+	0	0	0	0	0	+	0	+	0	+	+	0	+	+	+	0	+	0	+	+	+	+	0	+	0	2+		w
4	R0r	+	0	0	+	+	+	0	+	0	+	0	+	0	+	0	0	+	+	+	0	0	+	0	+	+	+	0	+	0	2+		w
5	r'r	0	+	0	+	+	+	0	0	0	+	0	+	0	+	0	+	+	0	+	+	0	0	+	+	0	+	0	+	0	0	2+	0
6	r''r	0	0	+	+	+	+	0	0	0	+	0	+	0	+	+	+	+	0	0	0	+	+	+	+	+	+	0	+	0	0	2+	0
7	rr	0	0	0	+	+	+	0	0	+	+	0	+	0	+	+	+	+	0	+	0	0	0	+	+	+	+	0	+	0	0	2+	0
8	rr	0	0	0	+	+	+	0	0	0	+	0	+	0	+	+	+	0	+	+	+	0	+	+	+	0	0	0	+	0	3+		1+
9	rr	0	0	0	+	+	+	0	0	0	+	0	+	0	+	+	0	+	+	0	0	+	+	+	0	+	0	0	+	0	2+		w
10	rr	0	0	0	+	+	+	0	0	0	+	0	+	0	+	+	+	+	+	0	0	+	+	0	+	0	0	0	+	0	2+		w
11	R1R1	+	+	0	0	+	0	0	0	+	+	0	+	0	+	0	+	+	0	+	0	+	0	+	0	+	0	0	+	0	0	2+	0
AC																														0	1+		

w: weak

7. Explain the difference in strength of reaction between cells 1, 2, and 8 and cells 3, 4, 9, and 10.

8. What is the most likely antibody identified by the antibody panel in Figure 1–8?

9. How would you rule out the remaining antibodies?

An elution was performed on Jane's RBCs with the following results on the last wash:

	AHG	CC
Screening Cell I	0	2+
Screening Cell II	0	2+

10. Do the reactions of the eluate confirm the antibody identified in question 6?

11. What type of transfusion reaction is illustrated by this case? What other antibodies are associated with this type of transfusion reaction?

12. Why is the transfusion history so important in working up any type and cross?

13. What other tests would provide useful information in this case? Explain why, and indicate the probable results.

RECOMMENDED READINGS

American Association of Blood Banks. (1999). *Technical Manual.* 13th ed. Bethesda, Md.: AABB.

Blaney, Kathy D. & Howard, Paula R. (2000). *Basic and Applied Concepts of Immunohematology.* St. Louis: Mosby.

Harmening, Denise M. (Ed.). (1999). *Modern Blood Banking and Transfusion Practices.* 4th ed. Philadelphia: F. A. Davis.

Quinley, Eva D. (1998). *Immunohematology: Principles and Practice.* 2nd ed. Philadelphia: J. B. Lippincott.

BLOOD BANK CASE 1–7*

Barbara J., a 30-year-old woman, delivered a healthy 6-lb, 3-oz baby girl at 39 weeks. A cord sample was sent to the blood bank on delivery. Approximately 24 hours after delivery, the blood bank received a request to perform a "type and Coombs" on the baby, who appeared jaundiced. The baby's blood had been tested, and the total bilirubin was 15.4 mg/dL. The blood bank results follow:

Forward Type		Reverse Type		Rh Typing		Direct Antiglobulin Test
Anti-A	Anti-B	A Cells	B Cells	Anti-D	D Control	
3+	0	NT	NT	0	0	1+

Abbreviation: NT, not tested.

On admission, a type and screen was performed on the mother. The results follow:

Forward Type		Reverse Type		Rh Typing	
Anti-A	Anti-B	A Cells	B Cells	Anti-D	D Control
0	0	3+	3+	4+	0

ANTIBODY SCREEN

	Screening Cell I				Screening Cell II				Screening Cell III				Autocontrol			
	IS	37	AHG	CC	IS	37	AHG	CC	IS	37	AHG	CC	IS	37	AHG	CC
Barbara J.	0	0	0	3+	0	0	0	3+	0	0	0	3+	0	0	0	2+

Follow-up Testing

A heat elution was performed on the baby's cells. The eluate was tested using A_1 and B cells at antihuman globulin phase. The results follow:

A_1 Cells	B Cells
1+	0

QUESTIONS

1. What is the most likely cause for the increase in the baby's bilirubin? Why?

* Data and sample questions courtesy of Ellen O. LaChance, M.S., M.T. (ASCP), S.B.B., Supervisor of Transfusion Service, Affiliated Laboratory/Eastern Maine Medical Center, Bangor, Maine.

2. Define genotype and phenotype.

3. What is the mother's ABO and Rh(D) genotype? What is the baby's ABO phenotype and Rh(D) genotype?

4. Could this condition have been predicted with prenatal testing performed on the mother?

5. Why was the baby's reverse grouping not performed?

6. What are the three major categories of this condition?

7. Which category does this case fall into? Why? Can it affect first pregnancies?

8. Why is this condition found primarily in group O mothers and group A babies?

9. What class of immunoglobulin is the antibody? Why?

10. Why is the eluate testing performed using antihuman globulin?

11. Should a fetal screen/Kleihauer-Betke be performed? Is the mother a candidate for Rhogam ($RH_0[D]$ immune globulin)? Why or why not?

12. What additional tests can be performed to confirm?

13. What treatment options are available?

14. Can anything be done to prevent this from happening in future pregnancies?

15. Should all cord bloods be tested by the blood bank?

RECOMMENDED READINGS

American Association of Blood Banks. (1999). *Technical Manual.* 13th ed. Bethesda, Md.: AABB.

Blaney, Kathy D. & Howard, Paula R. (2000). *Basic and Applied Concepts of Immunohematology.* St. Louis: Mosby.

Harmening, Denise M. (Ed.). (1999). *Modern Blood Banking and Transfusion Practices.* 4th ed. Philadelphia: F. A. Davis.

Quinley, Eva D. (1998). *Immunohematology: Principles and Practice.* 2nd ed. Philadelphia: J. B. Lippincott.

BLOOD BANK CASE 1-8

PATIENT 1

Anne L., a 48-year-old woman (5 ft 4 in, 125 lb), reported to her gynecologist that she had been extremely tired, physically weak, and did not have the energy to do her job. Upon questioning, she noted having very heavy menstrual periods lasting for 1 1/2 to 2 weeks. Her hemoglobin was 6.1 g/L; hematocrit, .19L/L; MCV (mean corpuscular volume), 70 fL; MCHC (mean corpuscular hemoglobin concentration), 27 g/dL.

1. Does Anne need a transfusion? Explain why or why not.

2. Support the viewpoint opposite to the one you expressed in question 1. Give a reason why a physician would take this stand.

3. What type of anemia is indicated by Anne's complete blood count (CBC) and medical history?

4. If Anne is transfused, what would be the recommended component and how many?

5.   a. If she is transfused with 3 U of packed cells, what would you estimate her hemoglobin and hematocrit to be following transfusion?

b. Would you expect the elevation to be slightly higher or lower than normal based on her size?

PATIENT 2

Carl M., a 50-year-old man, was scheduled for a colon resection. The preop orders included a CBC and crossmatch for 2 U. The CBC report was white blood cells (WBCs), 14.5×10^9/L; hemoglobin, 140 g/L; hematocrit, .43L/L; platelet count, 19,000/μL. The blood bank technologist typed him as O positive and cross-matched 2 U of O-positive packed cells.

6. Is additional component therapy other than the 2-U crossmatch indicated? Why?

7. How many units of the second component should be ordered?

8. Calculate the approximate platelet count following transfusion, assuming a 70-kg man.

9.   a. If Carl's 1-hour post-transfusion platelet count is 40,000/μL, what is his corrected count increment (CCI)? (Assume a body surface area of 1.5 m².)

     b. Is it normal, higher, or lower than expected?

     c. What does this indicate?

10. What are the storage temperature and shelf-life of platelets?

PATIENT 3

Melissa G., a 20-year-old woman who had been diagnosed with von Willebrand's disease, was scheduled for elective surgery. Her physician wanted to stabilize her von Willebrand's factor (vWF) before surgery and ordered a therapeutic trial of 1-deamino-8-D-arginine vasopressin (DDAVP) (Stimate [desmopressin]), a non-blood treatment that increases the release of vWF from storage sites (endothelial lining of blood vessels). She was a weak responder, and her vWF levels did not increase adequately; therefore, the next option was to use blood component therapy. Melissa had approximately 20% of the normal concentration of vWF.

11. What would you expect Melissa's results to be on the following coagulation tests (increased, normal, or decreased)?

   a. Prothrombin time (PT)

   b. Activated partial thromboplastin time (APTT)

   c. Platelet count

   d. Bleeding time

   e. VIII:C

   f. Ristocetin-induced platelet aggregation (RIPA)

12. Why did the physician try nonblood treatment before ordering blood component replacement therapy?

13. What is/are the component(s) of choice for stabilizing the concentration of vWF?

RECOMMENDED READINGS

American Association of Blood Banks. (1999). *Technical Manual.* 13th ed. Bethesda, Md.: AABB.

Blaney, Kathy D. & Howard, Paula R. (2000). *Basic and Applied Concepts of Immunohematology.* St. Louis: Mosby.

Harmening, Denise M. (Ed.). (1997). *Clinical Hematology and Fundamentals of Hemostasis.* 3rd ed. Philadelphia: F. A. Davis.

Harmening, Denise M. (Ed.). (1999). *Modern Blood Banking and Transfusion Practices.* 4th ed. Philadelphia: F. A. Davis.

Quinley, Eva D. (1998). *Immunohematology: Principles and Practice.* 2nd ed. Philadelphia: J. B. Lippincott.

BLOOD BANK CASE 1–9

Pat L., a 50-year-old woman, was admitted to the hospital for a hysterectomy. She had been transfused with 2 U of blood the previous year without incident. Her physician sent down orders for a 4-U crossmatch. Pat was A positive with a negative antibody screen. Four units of A positive were crossmatched by the blood bank technologist and found compatible.

The following morning, Pat was transfused with 2 U during surgery. Later that evening, Pat developed a temperature of 101°F and complained of chills. The evening technologist performed a transfusion reaction workup.

Clerical Errors

No clerical errors were found. Identification of patient and donor were confirmed.

	Pretransfusion Specimen	Post-transfusion Specimen
Hemolysis—urine	None detected	None detected
Hemolysis—serum	None detected	None detected
Direct antiglobulin test (DAT)	Negative	Negative

ANTIBODY SCREEN—PRETRANSFUSION

	Screening Cell I				Screening Cell II				Screening Cell III				Autocontrol			
	IS	37	AHG	CC	IS	37	AHG	CC	IS	37	AHG	CC	IS	37	AHG	CC
Pat L.	0	0	0	3+	0	0	0	3+	0	0	0	3+	0	0	0	2+

ANTIBODY SCREEN—POST-TRANSFUSION

	Screening Cell I				Screening Cell II				Screening Cell III				Autocontrol			
	IS	37	AHG	CC	IS	37	AHG	CC	IS	37	AHG	CC	IS	37	AHG	CC
Pat L.	0	0	0	3+	0	0	0	3+	0	0	0	3+	0	0	0	3+

QUESTIONS

1. Do Pat's laboratory test results indicate any evidence of in vitro hemolysis? Why or why not?

2. Does Pat have any alloantibodies and/or autoantibodies?

3. Did Pat have a transfusion reaction? If yes, what type of reaction is most likely?

4. What symptoms are associated with this condition?

5. Briefly describe two possible causes for this condition. How often does this occur; in other words, in what percentage of transfusions?

6. List five questions or bits of information about the patient that are useful when investigating this condition.

7.   a. Is this condition life-threatening?

      b. What other conditions may present a similar picture early on and must be ruled out?

8. How can this be prevented in the future?

9. List two groups of patients who have an increased incidence of this condition.

10. If any checks and procedures performed on this patient had been positive, what additional tests may be indicated?

RECOMMENDED READINGS

American Association of Blood Banks. (1999). *Technical Manual*. 13th ed. Bethesda, Md.: AABB.

Blaney, Kathy D. & Howard, Paula R. (2000). *Basic and Applied Concepts of Immunohematology*. St. Louis: Mosby.

Harmening, Denise M. (Ed.). (1999). *Modern Blood Banking and Transfusion Practices*. 4th ed. Philadelphia: F. A. Davis.

Quinley, Eva D. (1998). *Immunohematology: Principles and Practice*. 2nd. ed. Philadelphia: J. B. Lippincott.

BLOOD BANK CASE 1–10*

Paul D., a 63-year-old man, was admitted with a hemoglobin and hematocrit of 62 g/L (reference range, 135 to 175 g/L) and .19 (reference range, .41 to .53 L/L), respectively. He exhibited symptoms of fatigue, dizziness on standing, weakness, and chest pain. His physician ordered a type and crossmatch for 2 U. Paul was O positive, and the following results were reported.

ANTIBODY SCREEN

	Screening Cell I				Screening Cell II				Screening Cell III				Crossmatch			
	IS	37	AHG	CC	IS	37	AHG	CC	IS	37	AHG	CC	IS	37	AHG	CC
Paul D.	0	0	3+		0	0	3+		0	0	3+					
Unit 1													0	0	3+	
Unit 2													0	0	3+	

QUESTIONS

1. What additional testing is indicated?

DIRECT ANTIGLOBULIN TEST

	Paul D.	CC
Polyspecific AHG	2+	
Anti-IgG	2+	
Anti-C3	0	2+

2. What is the most probable explanation for this antibody problem?

* Data and sample questions courtesy of Ellen O. LaChance, M.S., M.T. (ASCP), S.B.B., Supervisor of Transfusion Service, Affiliated Laboratory/Eastern Maine Medical Center, Bangor, Maine.

3. List at least five conditions that have been associated with this group of antibodies.

4. How would you resolve this problem? What three pieces of information would you need in order to determine how to proceed?

Paul's blood bank results were reviewed, and the patient and his family w e interviewed. He had no record of a recent transfusion; therefore, a warm auto -sorption was performed. An antibody ID was then performed on the wa n autoabsorbed serum. The results are reported in Figure 1–9, "Antibody Panel, C e 1–10."

5.   a. Define absorption.

    b. What is the difference between warm autoabsorption and differen al (allogenic) absorption?

    c. When is allogenic absorption used?

Figure 1–9. ANTIBODY PANEL, CASE 1–10

No.	Rh	Rhesus								Kell						Duffy		Kidd		Sex Linked	Lewis		MNS				P	Lutheran		LISS		CC
		D	C	E	c	e	f	Cw	V	K	k	Kpa	Kpb	Jsa	Jsb	Fya	Fyb	Jka	Jkb	Xga	Lea	Leb	S	s	M	N	P1	Lua	Lub	37	AHG	CC
1	R1R1	+	+	0	0	+	0	+	0	0	+	0	+	0	+	+	0	+	+	0	0	+	0	+	+	+	0	0	+	0	0	2+
2	R1R1	+	+	0	0	+	0	0	0	0	+	0	+	0	+	+	+	0	+	+	+	0	+	+	+	+	+	0	+	0	0	2+
3	R2R2	+	0	+	+	0	0	0	0	0	+	+	+	0	+	0	+	+	+	0	0	+	+	0	+	0	+	0	+	0	0	2+
4	R0r	+	0	0	+	+	+	0	+	0	+	0	+	+	+	0	0	+	0	+	0	0	0	+	+	+	+	0	+	0	3+	
5	r'r	0	+	0	+	+	+	0	0	+	+	0	+	0	+	+	0	+	+	+	+	0	+	+	+	+	+	0	+	0	0	2+
6	r''r	0	0	+	+	+	+	0	0	0	+	0	+	0	+	+	0	+	+	0	0	+	0	+	+	+	+	0	+	0	3+	
7	rr	0	0	0	+	+	+	0	+	+	+	0	+	0	+	0	+	+	+	+	0	+	+	+	0	+	0	+	+	0	0	2+
8	rr	0	0	0	+	+	+	0	0	0	+	0	+	0	+	+	0	0	+	+	0	+	+	+	+	+	+	0	+	0	0	2+
9	rr	0	0	0	+	+	+	0	0	0	+	0	+	0	+	+	+	0	+	+	+	0	+	0	+	0	+	0	+	0	0	2+
10	rr	0	0	0	+	+	+	0	0	0	+	0	+	0	+	0	+	+	+	+	0	0	+	+	0	+	0	0	+	0	0	2+
11	R1R1	+	+	0	0	+	0	0	0	+	+	0	+	0	+	0	+	+	+	0	0	+	+	0	+	+	+	0	+	0	3	

w: weak

NT: not tested

6. What do the results indicate?

7. Does Paul have an underlying alloantibody(ies)? If so, what are they?

8.   a. What additional testing should be performed on the units cross-matched for this patient?

     b. What units should be crossmatched for this patient?

9. Will these units be compatible?

10. Will transfused RBCs have normal RBC survival?

RECOMMENDED READINGS

American Association of Blood Banks. (1999). *Technical Manual.* 13th ed. Bethesda, Md.: AABB.

Blaney, Kathy D. & Howard, Paula R. (2000). *Basic and Applied Concepts of Immunohematology.* St. Louis: Mosby.

Harmening, Denise M. (Ed.). (1999). *Modern Blood Banking and Transfusion Practices.* 4th ed. Philadelphia: F. A. Davis.

Quinley, Eva D. (1998). *Immunohematology: Principles and Practice.* 2nd ed. Philadelphia: J. B. Lippincott.

BLOOD BANK CASE 1–11

DONOR 1

Karen D., a 30-year-old female prospective donor, had the following relevant data from her physical examination and medical history:

Last donation:	6 months
Hemoglobin:	12.2 g/dL
Hematocrit:	37.0%
Pulse:	85 beats/min
Blood pressure:	150/80
Weight:	120
Temperature:	99.9°F

She had had her ears pierced with a second hole 4 months ago, and she was recovering from a cold.

1.   a. Do any of the values in the physical examination or answers to the questions in her medical history fall outside of the acceptable limits established by American Association of Blood Banks (AABB)? How many?

   b. If any, list the value or criteria and the acceptable limit.

2.   a. Would Karen be accepted, temporarily deferred, or permanently deferred?

b. If deferred for a certain period of time, how long?

3. Is the fact that Karen has a cold a reason for temporary deferral?

DONOR 2

Mike H., a 41-year-old male prospective donor, who was a college professor, presented with the following physical examination and medical history:

Last donation:	10 weeks ago
Hemoglobin:	13.4 g/dL
Hematocrit:	40.2%
Pulse:	78 beats/min
Blood pressure:	140/88
Weight:	165
Temperature:	98.8°F

He answered "Yes" to the question "In the last 12 months, have you had close contact with a person with jaundice or hepatitis?"

4.   a. Do any of the values in the physical examination or answers to the questions in the medical history fall outside of the acceptable limits established by AABB? How many?

b. If any, list the criteria and the acceptable limit.

5. What group is considered exempt from the question regarding "close contact with a person with jaundice or hepatitis"?

Upon further questioning, it was determined that Mike's wife had been diagnosed with hepatitis C 3 months ago.

6. a. Would Mike be accepted, temporarily deferred, or permanently deferred?

b. If deferred for a certain period of time, how long?

DONOR 3

Heidi M., an 18-year-old female prospective donor who was a college freshman, presented with the following physical examination and relevant questions from the medical history:

Last donation:	None, first-time donor
Hemoglobin:	13.0 g/dL

Hematocrit:	39.2%
Pulse:	105 beats/min
Blood pressure:	130/80
Weight:	124
Temperature:	98.5°F

She had been taking Acutane (isotretinoin) for acne but had taken her last dose 3 months ago.

7.   a. Do any of the values in the physical examination or answers to the questions in the medical history fall outside of the acceptable limits established by AABB? How many?

   b. If any, list the criteria and the acceptable limit.

8. What would you do next?

9.   a. Would Heidi be accepted, temporarily deferred, or permanently deferred?

b. If deferred for a certain period of time, how long?

RECOMMENDED READINGS

American Association of Blood Banks. (1999). *Technical Manual.* 13th ed. Bethesda, Md.: AABB.

Blaney, Kathy D. & Howard, Paula R. (2000). *Basic and Applied Concepts of Immunohematology.* St. Louis: Mosby.

Harmening, Denise M. (Ed.). (1999). *Modern Blood Banking and Transfusion Practices.* 4th ed. Philadelphia: F. A. Davis.

Quinley, Eva D. (1998). *Immunohematology: Principles and Practice.* 2nd ed. Philadelphia: J. B. Lippincott.

Chemistry

CHEMISTRY CASE 2–1

Linda D., a 13-year-old girl who was a known diabetic, became comatose and was rushed to the hospital by her parents. Two days before admission, she went to school feeling ill and vomited that evening. Linda's vomiting persisted with only a 6-hour pause during sleep. She refused to take her insulin the following morning, even after she had been instructed to give herself the regular insulin dose and control her nausea with Tigan (trimethobenzamide HCl). The emergency room (ER) physician noted that she was breathing deeply and rapidly and that her breath had a fruity odor. The laboratory results are shown in Tables 2–1 to 2–3.

■ Table 2–1 ■ CHEMISTRY

	Linda D.	Reference Range
Glucose	430	70–105 mg/dL
BUN	43	8–26 mg/dL
Creatinine	2.6	0.6–1.2 mg/dL
Sodium	129	136–145 mmol/L
Potassium	5.8	3.5–5.0 mmol/L
Chloride	88	99–109 mmol/L
Total CO_2	9	21–28 mmol/L
HCO_3	10	22–28 mmol/L
Cholesterol	525	Recommended (desirable): <200 mg/dL
Triglyceride	3800	Recommended (desirable): <250 mg/dL

Abbreviation: BUN, blood urea nitrogen.

■ Table 2–2 ■ URINALYSIS

	Linda D.	Reference Range
Macroscopic		
Color	Straw	Colorless to amber
Appearance	Clear	Clear
Specific gravity	1.014	1.001–1.035
pH	6.0	5–7
Protein	Neg	Neg

■ **Table 2–2** ■ **URINALYSIS** (continued)

	Linda D.	Reference Range
Macroscopic		
Glucose	3+	Neg
Ketones	3+	Neg
Bilirubin	Neg	Neg
Blood	Neg	Neg
Urobilinogen	Normal	Normal
Nitrite	Neg	Neg
Leukocyte esterase	Neg	Neg
Microscopic		
WBCs	0–2/HPF	0–5/HPF
RBCs	0–1/HPF	0–2/HPF
Epithelial cells	Few squamous/HPF	Few–moderate
Casts	Neg	Few hyaline
Bacteria	Neg	None

Abbreviations: HPF, high-power field; RBCs, red blood cells; WBCs, white blood cells.

(Handwritten margin note: Correlate with fruity odor breath)

■ **Table 2–3** ■ **COMPLETE BLOOD COUNT**

	Linda D.	Reference Range
WBC	11.0	$5–10 \times 10^9$/L
RBC	5.80	$4.0–5.0 \times 10^{12}$/L
Hb	154	120–160 g/L
Hct	.46	.36–.46 L/L
MCV	88	80–100 fL
MCH	29	26–34 pg
MCHC	35	31–37%
Platelets	357	$150–400 \times 10^9$/L
Segmented neutrophils	57	25–60%
Band	2	0–10%
Lymphocytes	32	20–50%
Monocytes	8	2–11%
Eosinophils	1	0–8%
Basophils	0	0–2%
Atypical lymphocytes	0	0–5%
RBC morphology	Normal	Normal

Abbreviations: MCH, mean corpuscular hemoglobin; MCHC, mean corpuscular hemoglobin (Hb) concentration; MCV, mean corpuscular volume.

QUESTIONS

1. What are the abnormal laboratory results?

2. What is Linda's clinical condition, and what caused the condition?

3. a. What is the typical blood gas profile in this acid–base imbalance?

    b. What triggered her abnormal breathing (deeply and rapidly)?

    c. What is giving the fruity odor to Linda's breath?

4. Why is the glucose elevated?

5. What type of diabetic is she? Explain why.

6. List the three major ketone bodies.

7. Which ketone body was *not* measured using the routine urinalysis reagent strip reaction?

8. Explain the electrolyte results.

9. Calculate the osmolality from the laboratory data. Is it increased, decreased, or normal?

10. What additional test could the physician order to calculate the patient's average glucose level for the past 6 to 8 weeks to determine the patient's compliance with diet and insulin recommendations?

11. What are two possible explanations for the elevated BUN and creatinine in this patient?

12.   a. Calculate the anion gap.

     b. What is the cause of this abnormal calculated anion gap?

13. Are the elevated cholesterol and triglyceride consistent with Linda's clinical picture?

RECOMMENDED READINGS

Anderson, Shauna C. & Cockayne, Susan. (1993). *Clinical Chemistry: Concepts and Applications.* Philadelphia: W. B. Saunders.

Bishop, Michael L., Duben-Engelkirk, Janet L. & Fody, Edward P. (2000). *Clinical Chemistry: Principles, Procedures Correlations.* 4th ed. Philadelphia: J. B. Lippincott.

Burtis, Carl A. & Ashwood, Edward R. (1999). *Tietz Textbook of Clinical Chemistry.* 3rd ed. Philadelphia: W. B. Saunders.

Burtis, Carl A. & Ashwood, Edward R. (Eds.). (2001). *Tietz Fundamentals of Clinical Chemistry.* 5th ed. Philadelphia: W. B. Saunders.

Diabetes Care: Standards of Medical Care for Patients with Diabetes Mellitus. (1999). [On-line] Available: www.diabetes.org/DiabetesCare/Supplement199/S32.htm [1999, March 29].

Lehman, Craig A. (1998). *Saunders Manual of Clinical Laboratory Science.* Philadelphia: W. B. Saunders.

CHEMISTRY CASE 2–2

Kathy T., a 60-year-old woman, was seen in the ER complaining of chest pain, which was moderate to severe. She had experienced substernal pain for the previous 6 to 7 weeks with dyspnea on exertion. The pain, however, had become more frequent and severe, with constant pain and pressure for the last 2 to 3 days. Kathy appeared anxious and complained of weakness, sweating, and nausea. Her blood pressure was 110/66. Her laboratory results are shown in Tables 2–4 to 2–7.

■ Table 2–4 ■ CHEMISTRY RESULTS

	Day 1	Day 4	Day 6	Day 9	Day 11	Reference Range
Sodium	136	130	139	143	153	135–145 mEq/L
Potassium	3.7	3.0	4.3	3.9	3.8	3.6–5.0 mEq/L
Chloride	94	103	107	113	114	98–107 mEq/L
CO_2	—	25.0	24.0	23	30.0	24.0–34.0 mEq/L
Anion gap	—	2.0	8.0	7.0	9.0	10–20 mmol/L
Glucose	319	519	379	310	234	80–120 mg/dL
BUN	23	53	81	99	79	7–24 mg/dL
Creatinine	0.9	1.4	2.3	2	1.9	0.5–1.2 mg/dL
Calcium	9.7	—	—	—	—	8.5–10.5 mg/dL
Magnesium	—	1.1	1.7	1.9	2.0	1.3–2.5 mEq/L
Digoxin	—	—	2.60	1.12	—	0.80–2.00 ng/mL
Cholesterol	350	—	—	—	—	0–200 mg/dL
Triglyceride	275	—	—	—	—	10–190 mg/dL
Bilirubin	0.2	—	—	—	—	0.2–1.2 mg/dL
AST	76	—	—	—	—	5–40 IU/L
ALP	84	—	—	—	—	30–157 IU/L
Total protein	7.3	—	—	—	—	6.0–8.4 g/dL
Albumin	4.1	—	—	—	—	3.5–5.0 g/dL
TSH	—	—	—	0.72	—	0.49–4.67 µIU/mL

Abbreviations: ALP, alkaline phosphatase; AST, aspartate aminotransferase; TSH, thyroid-stimulating hormone.

■ Table 2–5 ■ BLOOD GAS

	Day 2	Reference Range
Arterial pH	7.20	7.35–7.45
PCO_2	63.7	35.0–45.0 mm Hg
PO_2	64.0	75.0–85.0 mm Hg
HCO_3^-	25.4	20.0–25.0 mmol/L
TCO_2	27.4	21.0–27.0 mmol/L
Base excess	-3.3	-3.0–3.0 mmol/L
% Saturated	86	

Abbreviations: PCO_2, partial pressure of carbon dioxide; PO_2, partial pressure of oxygen; TCO_2, total CO_2.

■ Table 2–6 ■   CARDIAC PROFILE

	Day 1	Day 2	Day 2	Day 2	Day 3	Day 4	Reference Range
Time	20:30	5:06	12:25	20:35	12:15	7:15	
CK	668	1383	3461	3743	2117	973	24–170 IU/L
CK-MB	47.1	NT	146.6	93.0	24.8	12.1	0.0–3.8 ng/mL
Troponin I	36.6	184.0	5745.0	926.1	NT	NT	0.0–0.4 ng/mL

CK-MB Reference Range		Troponin I Reference Range
0–3.8:	Normal	0–0.4 ng/mL: No evidence of myocardial injury
3.9–10.4:	Borderline	0.5–2.0 ng/mL: Mild elevation, suggesting possible myocardial injury
>10.4:	Significantly elevated	>2.0 ng/mL: Significantly elevated, consistent with myocardial injury

Abbreviations: CK, creatine kinase; NT, not tested.

Kathy was given Nitrostat (nitroglycerine tablets) 1/150 grain prn for pain, and Inderal (propranolol HCl) was administered. She was also taking digoxin. The electrocardiogram (ECG) was performed and revealed an atrial flutter and the possibility of a true posterior infarct and lateral ischemia.

Her complete blood count (CBC) indicated a mild normocytic, normochromic anemia. The WBC was 16.4×10^9/L (reference range, $5–10 \times 10^9$/L) on the day following admission.

■ Table 2–7 ■   URINALYSIS

	Kathy T.	Reference Range
Macroscopic		
Color	Yellow	Colorless to amber
Appearance	Clear	Clear
Specific gravity	1.018	1.001–1.035
pH	6.0	5–7
Protein	Neg	Neg
Glucose	2+	Neg
Ketones	Trace	Neg
Bilirubin	Neg	Neg
Blood	Neg	Neg
Urobilinogen	Normal	Normal
Nitrite	Neg	Neg
Leukocyte esterase	Neg	Neg
Microscopic		
WBCs	0–2/HPF	0–5/HPF
RBCs	0–1/HPF	0–2/HPF
Epithelial cells	Few squamous/HPF	Few to moderate
Casts	Neg	Few hyaline
Bacteria	Neg	None

Abbreviation: HPF, high-power field.

QUESTIONS

1. After reading Kathy's initial patient history, what chemistry profile would the ER physician order on this patient? What tests are included in this profile in your laboratory, and what are the collection times?

2. What laboratory results in Tables 2–4 to 2–6 are abnormal?

3. The laboratory results in Tables 2–4 and 2–6 indicate what condition? Explain briefly (2 to 3 sentences) the pathogenesis (the process).

4. Heart muscle contains which CK isoenzyme(s)?

5. How many hours after a myocardial infarction would you find an elevated CK and CK-MB? How long would they remain elevated?

6. Define CK relative index (RI). Calculate the CK-MB RI for all specimens with total CK and CK-MB.

7. How many hours postinfarction would you find elevated cardiac troponin I and cardiac troponin T, and how long would they remain elevated?

8. What is the difference in *specificity* for myocardial damage between cardiac troponin I and cardiac troponin T?

9. What is the cause of the elevated AST?

10. What other chemistry test(s) have been developed that could be included in a cardiac profile?

11. What acute reaction protein is rapidly gaining acceptance as an indicator of increased risk for AMI and stroke?

12. What other medical problem/condition does this patient have? What laboratory values support your decision?

13. Do patients with the condition you described in the previous questions have a higher risk of myocardial infarction or stroke than the general population? Why or why not?

14. Is the elevated WBC consistent with Kathy's condition?

RECOMMENDED READINGS

Bishop, Michael L., Duben-Engelkirk, Janet L. & Fody, Edward P. (2000). *Clinical Chemistry: Principles, Procedures Correlations*. 4th ed. Philadelphia: J. B. Lippincott.

Burtis, Carl A. & Ashwood, Edward R. (2001). *Tietz Fundamentals of Clinical Chemistry*. 5th ed. Philadelphia: W. B. Saunders.

Damjanov, Ivan. (1996). *Pathology for the Health-Related Professions*. Philadelphia: W. B. Saunders.

Davis, Brenta G., Bishop, Michael L. & Mass, Diana (Eds.). (1989). *Clinical Laboratory Science: Strategies for Practice*. Philadelphia: J. B. Lippincott.

Jaffe, Allan. (1998). *Ruling Out Myocardial Infarction with Serologic Markers*. [On-line] Available: www.medscape.com/medscape/CNO/1998/ACC/04.01/acc0708.jaff/acc0708.jaff.html

Lehman, Craig A. (1998). *Saunders Manual of Clinical Laboratory Science*. Philadelphia: W. B. Saunders.

National Academy of Clinical Biochemistry. (1998). *Use of Cardiac Markers in Coronary Artery Disease*. [On-line] Available: www.nacb.org/nacb_SOLP_ [1998, October 6].

CHEMISTRY CASE 2–3

Jane L., a 30-year-old woman, was seen in the ER with severe epigastric pain radiating to the back that woke her from sleep. She also complained of nausea and vomiting. The chemistry and hematology tests shown in Tables 2–8 and 2–9 were ordered.

■ Table 2–8 ■ CHEMISTRY TESTS

	Jane L.	Reference Range
Sodium	140	135–145 mEq/L
Potassium	3.6	3.6–5.0 mEq/L
Chloride	106	98–107 mEq/L
CO_2	29.0	24.0–34.0 mEq/L
Glucose	116	80–120 mg/dL
Bilirubin, total	0.2	0.2–1.9 mg/dL
AST	26	5–40 IU/L
ALP	53	30–157 IU/L
Protein	6.8	6.0–8.4 g/dL

	2/20	2/21	Reference Range
BUN	13	14	7–24 mg/dL
Creatinine	1.2	1.2	0.5–1.2 mg/dL
Calcium	9.0	8.8	8.5–10.5 mg/dL
Albumin	4.2	NT	3.5–5.0 g/dL
ALT	23	NT	5–40 IU/L
Amylase	738	265	10–110 IU/L
Lipase	3970*	320	31–186 IU/L
γGT	335	NT	13–86 IU/L
Cholesterol	NT	165	Recommended (desirable): < 200 mg/dL
Triglyceride	NT	155	Recommended (desirable): < 250 mg/dL
HDL	NT	35	Recommended (desirable): ≥ 60 mg/dL
LDL	NT	99	Recommended (desirable): ≤ 130 mg/dL

*Lipemic sample, results rechecked.
Abbreviations: ALT, alanine aminotransferase; γGT, gamma glutamyltransferase; HDL, high-density lipoprotein; LDL, low-density lipoprotein; NT, not tested.

■ Table 2–9 ■ HEMATOLOGY

	2/20	2/21	Reference Range
WBC	12.1	10.8	$5-10 \times 10^9$/L
RBC	4.93	4.76	$4.0-5.0 \times 10^{12}$/L
ESR	40	NT	0–20 mm/h

Abbreviations: ESR, erythrocyte sedimentation rate; NT, not tested.

QUESTIONS

1. Circle or highlight the abnormal laboratory values.

2.   a. Jane's profile is indicative of what condition?

      b. Briefly describe the pathogenesis involved (origin and development of disease).

3.   a. What are the two most common causes/etiologies of this condition?

      b. List three other less common causes.

4. Which two enzymes are critical in the diagnosis of this disease? Discuss the typical enzyme activity curve (elevation, peak, return to normal), sensitivity, and specificity of these enzymes.

5. List five other causes for an elevated amylase. How can they be differentiated from acute pancreatitis?

6. Discuss the significance of the other abnormal tests.

7. Why would a physician order a urine amylase/creatinine ratio on a patient with elevated amylase?

8.   a. What factors (use Ranson's prognostic signs; see Lehman, 1998) are used to assess the severity and prognosis of this disease?

b. Based on the information you have, does this patient have any of the signs indicating a more serious prognosis?

9. List and briefly describe four important local complications of this disease, including the cause of the complication (why it occurs).

10. What is the usual course of treatment?

REFERENCE

Lehman, Craig A. (1998). *Saunders Manual of Clinical Laboratory Science.* Philadelphia: W. B. Saunders.

RECOMMENDED READINGS

Bishop, Michael L., Duben-Engelkirk, Janet L. & Fody, Edward P. (2000). *Clinical Chemistry: Principles, Procedures Correlations.* 4th ed. Philadelphia: J. B. Lippincott.

Burtis, Carl A. & Ashwood, Edward R. (1996). *Tietz Fundamentals of Clinical Chemistry*. 4th ed. Philadelphia: W. B. Saunders.

Burtis, Carl A. & Ashwood, Edward R. (1999). *Tietz Textbook of Clinical Chemistry*. 3rd ed. Philadelphia: W. B. Saunders.

Damjanov, Ivan. (1996). *Pathology for the Health-Related Professions*. Philadelphia: W. B. Saunders.

Love, Jonathan. (2000). *Open for Discussion: Acute Pancreatitis*. [On-line] Available: www.cag-acg.org/sponsors/janssen/open_for_discussion/case25/case25.html.

CHEMISTRY CASE 2–4

Tom N., a 60-year-old man, came into the ER complaining of fatigue and overall flulike symptoms. He was mildly jaundiced with icteric sclera. His liver profile and CBC results are shown in Tables 2–10 and 2–11.

■ Table 2–10 ■   LIVER PROFILE

	2/15	2/22	Reference Range
Bilirubin, total	2.2	1.9	0.2–1.2 mg/dL
Bilirubin, direct	1.19	NT	0.00–0.40 mg/dL
AST	564	735	5–40 IU/L
ALP	202	NT	30–157 IU/L
ALT	373	NT	5–40 IU/L
Albumin	2.1	1.9	3.5–5.0 g/dL
Total protein	7.4	7.4	6.0–8.4 g/dL
Ammonia	32	48	20–80 µg/dL
Folic acid	17.8	NT	2.9–15.6 ng/dL
Vitamin B$_{12}$	377	NT	180–710 pg/mL

Abbreviation: NT, not tested.

■ Table 2–11 ■   COMPLETE BLOOD COUNT

	Tom N.	Reference Range
WBC	2.1	5–10×10^9/L
RBC	4.10	5–6×10^{12}/L
Hb	138	135–175 g/L
Hct	.39	.41–.53 L/L
MCV	97	80–100 fL
MCH	33	26–34 pg
MCHC	35	31–37%
Platelets	42	150–400×10^9/L
Segmented neutrophils	69	25–60%
Lymphocytes	16	20–50%
Monocytes	10	2–11%
Eosinophils	4	0–8%
Basophils	1	0–2%
RBC morphology	Normal	Normal

QUESTIONS

1. Circle or highlight the abnormal results in Tables 2–10 and 2–11.

2. What organ system is involved?

3. List six probable explanations for this chemistry profile.

4. What is the most likely explanation for these results?

Hepatitis Serum Panel

IgM anti-HAV:	Nonreactive
HBsAg:	Nonreactive
IgM anti-HBc:	Nonreactive
Anti-HCV:	Reactive

5. What is the most likely diagnosis for this patient?

6. List five main etiologic factors (causes) for this infection.

7. List at least six groups who have a higher than normal risk of infection (high-risk groups)?

8.   a. Calculate the De Ritis ratio.

     b. What does it indicate in this patient?

9. Describe the pathogenesis (what happens).

10. How can the physician differentiate between acute and chronic forms of this infection?

RECOMMENDED READINGS

Bishop, Michael L., Duben-Engelkirk, Janet L. & Fody, Edward P. (2000). *Clinical Chemistry: Principles, Procedures Correlations.* 4th ed. Philadelphia: J. B. Lippincott.

Burtis, Carl A. & Ashwood, Edward R. (1999). *Tietz Textbook of Clinical Chemistry.* 3rd ed. Philadelphia: W. B. Saunders.

Burtis, Carl A. & Ashwood, Edward R. (2001). *Tietz Fundamentals of Clinical Chemistry.* 5th ed. Philadelphia: W. B. Saunders.

Hepnet. (1999). *Initial Interferon Therapy Cost-Effective for Chronic Hepatitis C Patients.* [On-line] Available: hepnet.com/hepc/news122398.html [1999, February 2].

Kaplan, Lawrence A. & Pesce, Amadeo J. (1996). *Clinical Chemistry: Theory, Analysis, Correlation.* 3rd ed. St. Louis: Mosby.

Lehman, Craig A. (1998). *Saunders Manual of Clinical Laboratory Science.* Philadelphia: W. B. Saunders.

Niederu, Claus, Lange, Stefan, Heintges, Tobias, et al. (1999). *Prognosis of Chronic Hepatitis C: Results of a Large, Prospective Cohort Study.* [On-line] Available: www.hepatology.org./cgi.content/full/ [1999, February 3].

CHEMISTRY CASE 2–5

Bobby J., a 12-year-old boy, was seen in the ER complaining of fatigue, vague flu-like symptoms, and muscle pain in his legs. His laboratory results are shown in Tables 2–12 and 2–13.

■ Table 2–12 ■ CHEMISTRY

	Bobby J.	Reference Range
Bilirubin, total	0.3	0.2–1.2 mg/dL
Bilirubin, direct	0.08	0.00–0.40 mg/dL
AST	29	5–40 IU/L
ALP	550	60–500 IU/L
Albumin	3.9	3.5–5.0 g/dL
ALT	17	5–40 IU/L
γGT	29	5–45 IU/L
Calcium	11.0	8.5–10.5 mg/dL
Phosphate	5.1	2.7–4.5 mg/dL

■ Table 2–13 ■ COMPLETE BLOOD COUNT

	Bobby J.	Reference Range
WBC	7.8	$5–10 \times 10^9$/L
RBC	4.85	$5–6 \times 10^{12}$/L
Hb	140	140–180 g/L
Hct	.41	.41–.53 L/L
MCV	88	80–100 fL
MCH	30	26–34 pg
MCHC	34	31–37%
Platelets	204	$150–400 \times 10^9$/L
RDW	13.4	11.6–14.8%

Abbreviation: RDW, red blood cell distribution width index.

QUESTIONS

1. What laboratory values are abnormal?

2. What organ systems could be responsible for the increase?

3. Which organ systems can be ruled out because of other test results in the profile?

4. List four *possible* explanations for the abnormal result.

5. What is the *probable* explanation for the abnormal result?

6. Should the physician be concerned about the elevated calcium and phosphorous?

RECOMMENDED READINGS

Bishop, Michael L., Duben-Engelkirk, Janet L. & Fody, Edward P. (2000). *Clinical Chemistry: Principles, Procedures Correlations.* 4th ed. Philadelphia: J. B. Lippincott.

Burtis, Carl A. & Ashwood, Edward R. (2001). *Tietz Fundamentals of Clinical Chemistry.* 5th ed. Philadelphia: W. B. Saunders.

Burtis, Carl A. & Ashwood, Edward R. (1999). *Tietz Textbook of Clinical Chemistry.* 3rd ed. Philadelphia: W. B. Saunders.

Kaplan, Lawrence A. & Pesce, Amadeo J. (1996). *Clinical Chemistry: Theory, Analysis, Correlation.* 3rd ed. St. Louis: Mosby.

Lehman, Craig A. (1998). *Saunders Manual of Clinical Laboratory Science.* Philadelphia: W. B. Saunders.

CHEMISTRY CASE 2–6

Melissa R., a 25-year-old woman who was 6 months postpartum, visited her physician with complaints of tiredness, always feeling cold, muscle weakness, menorrhagia, and weight gain. Her physician noted some facial edema and dry skin. Melissa's CBC indicated a mild normocytic, normochromic anemia. See Tables 2–14 and 2–15.

■ Table 2–14 ■ CHEMISTRY RESULTS

	Melissa R.	Reference Range
Sodium	136	135–145 mEq/L
Potassium	3.7	3.6–5.0 mEq/L
Chloride	94	98–107 mEq/L
CO_2	30.0	24.0–34.0 mEq/L
Glucose	90	80–120 mg/dL
BUN	23	7–24 mg/dL
Creatinine	0.9	0.5–1.2 mg/dL
Calcium	9.7	8.5–10.5 mg/dL
Cholesterol	310	Recommended (desirable): <200 mg/dL
Triglyceride	200	Recommended (desirable): <250 mg/dL
Bilirubin	0.2	0.2–1.2 mg/dL
AST	40	5–40 IU/L
ALP	68	30–157 IU/L
CK	300	24–179 IU/L
Total protein	7.3	6.0–8.4 g/dL
Albumin	4.1	3.5–5.0 g/dL

■ Table 2–15 ■ THYROID PROFILE

	Melissa R.	Reference Range
TSH	21.896	0.300–5.000 µIU/mL
Total T_4	7.33	4.60–11.0 µg/dL
T_3 Uptake	26	25–30%
Free thyroxine index (FTI)	1.91	4.5–12

QUESTIONS

1. Circle or highlight Melissa's abnormal test results.

2. What is the most likely explanation for Melissa's results?

3. What are the two major categories or types of this disease/condition? List four causes under each type.

4.   a. Under which of the major categories would Melissa be classified?

      b. Why?

      c. Which test is used to rule out or rule in one of the major categories?

5. What subcategory (listed in question 4) would be the most likely explanation for this patient?

6. What test(s) are recommended to screen for this condition?

7. What does the T_3 uptake measure? List four nonthyroidal conditions associated with an increased T_3 uptake. List at least four nonthyroidal conditions associated with a decreased T_3 uptake.

8. List at least six common symptoms/signs of this disorder.

9. What other tests might be useful to determine Melissa's status? Why?

10. Are the elevated cholesterol, triglyceride, and CK consistent with this diagnosis?

RECOMMENDED READINGS

Bishop, Michael L., Duben-Engelkirk, Janet L. & Fody, Edward P. (2000). *Clinical Chemistry: Principles, Procedures Correlations.* 4th ed. Philadelphia: J. B. Lippincott.

Burtis, Carl A. & Ashwood, Edward R. (1999). *Tietz Textbook of Clinical Chemistry.* 3rd ed. Philadelphia: W. B. Saunders.

Burtis, Carl A. & Ashwood, Edward R. (2001). *Tietz Fundamentals of Clinical Chemistry.* 5th ed. Philadelphia: W. B. Saunders.

Kaplan, Lawrence A. & Pesce, Amadeo J. (1996). *Clinical Chemistry: Theory, Analysis, Correlation.* 3rd ed. St. Louis: Mosby.

Lehman, Craig A. (1998). *Saunders Manual of Clinical Laboratory Science.* Philadelphia: W. B. Saunders.

Wiersinga, W. M. & DeGroot, Leslie J. (1999). "*Chapter 9. Adult Hypothyroidism.*" [On-line] Available: www.thyroidmanager.org/Chapter9/9-text.htm [2000, July 5].

CHEMISTRY CASE 2–7

Phil C., a 76-year-old man, was admitted through the ER with difficulty breathing, coughing, and chest pain. See Table 2–16.

■ Table 2–16 ■ CHEMISTRY RESULTS

	2/18	2/19	Reference Range
Sodium	141	140	136–145 mEq/L
Potassium	4.4	4.7	3.6–5.0 mEq/L
Chloride	107	106	101–111 mEq/L
CO_2	27.0	30.0	24.0–34.0 mEq/L
Anion gap	5.0	5.0	10–20 mmol/L
Glucose	95	112	80–120 mg/dL
Bilirubin, total	0.3	NT	0.2–1.2 mg/dL
Troponin I	<0.3	<0.3	0.0–0.4 ng/mL
AST	10	NT	5–40 IU/L
ALP	42	NT	30–157 IU/L
Protein	6.5	NT	6.0–8.4 g/dL
BUN	53	49	7–24 mg/dL
Creatinine	2.0	1.8	0.5–1.2 mg/dL
Calcium	8.8	NT	8.5–10.5 mg/dL
Albumin	3.6	NT	3.5–5.0 g/dL
Digoxin	1.06	0.82	0.00–2.00 ng/mL
CK	100	NT	24–170 IU/L
CK-MB	3.1	3.2	*

*0–3.8 ng/mL = normal; 3.9–10.4 = borderline; >10.4 = significantly elevated.
Abbreviation: NT, not tested.

QUESTIONS

1. What are Phil's abnormal test results?

2. Do the laboratory results rule out a myocardial infarction?

3. What is Phil's BUN/creatinine ratio? What is a normal BUN/creatinine ratio?

4. What type of azotemia does this indicate?

5.   a. What are some of the causes of this type of azotemia?

     b. List five conditions associated with this type of azotemia.

6. What is the most likely diagnosis in this case?

7. What is digoxin? Is it associated with Phil's condition?

8. What is congestive heart failure (CHF)?

9. List five common risk factors for CHF.

RECOMMENDED READINGS

Bishop, Michael L., Duben-Engelkirk, Janet L. & Fody, Edward P. (2000). *Clinical Chemistry: Principles, Procedures Correlations.* 4th ed. Philadelphia: J. B. Lippincott.

Burtis, Carl A. & Ashwood, Edward R. (1999). *Tietz Textbook of Clinical Chemistry.* 3rd ed. Philadelphia: W. B. Saunders.

Burtis, Carl A. & Ashwood, Edward R. (2001). *Tietz Fundamentals of Clinical Chemistry.* 5th ed. Philadelphia: W. B. Saunders.

HealthAnswers. (1999). [On-line] Available: www.healthanswers.com/ Cente...w.asp?id=heart&filename=000158.htm [2000, February 24].

Kaplan, Lawrence A. & Pesce, Amadeo J. (1996). *Clinical Chemistry: Theory, Analysis, Correlation.* 3rd ed. St. Louis: Mosby.

Lehman, Craig A. (1998). *Saunders Manual of Clinical Laboratory Science.* Philadelphia: W. B. Saunders.

Life Extension Foundation. (1999). [On-line] Available: www.lef.org/protocols/ prtcl-037.shtml [2000, February 25].

CHEMISTRY CASE 2–8

Brian H., an 80-year-old man with a history of chronic obstructive pulmonary disease (COPD) and respiratory infections, was admitted through the ER with a chronic cough and extreme dyspnea (extreme respiratory distress). He complained that he was unable to climb stairs or anything else that required any exertion (even washing his hair). He had been a heavy smoker but had been attempting to stop smoking by cutting back on the number of cigarettes per day. The nurse noted his temperature was 101.2°F. See Tables 2–17 and 2–18.

■ Table 2–17 ■   ARTERIAL BLOOD GAS RESULTS ON ADMISSION

	Brian H.	Reference Range
pH	7.230	7.35–7.45
PCO_2	75.0	35–45 mm Hg
PO_2	28.2	83–108 mm Hg
HCO_3^-	32.7	22–28 mEq/L
SaO_2	49.6	95–98%
COHb	8.6	Nonsmokers: 0.5–1.5%
		Smokers:
		1–2 packs/day: 4–5%
		> 2 packs/day: 8–9%

Abbreviations: COHb, carboxyhemoglobin; PCO_2, partial pressure of carbon dioxide; PO_2, partial pressure of oxygen; SaO_2, oxygen saturation, arterial.

QUESTIONS

1. What are the abnormal blood gas values?

2. What is Brian's acid–base status (normal, acidosis, or alkalosis)?

3. Is the condition that is responsible for the blood gases respiratory, metabolic/nonrespiratory, or mixed? Explain.

4. Is the condition acute or chronic? In other words, is it uncompensated, partially compensated, or fully compensated? Why?

5. a. What is the primary compensatory mechanism in this acid–base disorder?

   b. List three processes it uses to compensate for the imbalance.

   c. What other system is responsible for compensatory mechanisms in acid–base disorders? How does it compensate?

    d. Why is it often inefficient in this acid–base disorder?

6. Would the oxyhemoglobin dissociation curve be shifted? If yes, what direction (right or left)? And explain why.

7. Briefly describe base excess and base deficit. Would this patient have a base excess, base deficit, or normal base?

8. What level of HCO_3^- would compensate for the increased PCO_2 and correct the pH to normal?

9. What conditions are associated with this acid–base disorder?

10. Which condition is the most likely explanation in this case?

11. A deficiency of what protein is associated with a family history of this condition?

12. What is the probable cause of the elevated temperature?

13. Briefly discuss what is meant by COPD.

Six hours later, the arterial blood gases (ABGs) in Table 2–18 were reported.

■ Table 2–18 ■ ABG RESULTS 6 HOURS POSTADMISSION

	Brian H.	Reference Range
pH	7.38	7.35–7.45
PCO_2	60.0	35–45 mm Hg
PO_2	78.2	83–108 mm Hg
HCO_3^-	36.2	22–28 mEq/L
SaO_2	90.6	95–98%
COHb	3.6	Nonsmokers: 0.5–1.5%
		Smokers:
		1–2 packs/day: 4–5%
		> 2 packs/day: 8–9%

14. What is Brian's acid–base status at this point?

RECOMMENDED READINGS

Bishop, Michael L., Duben-Engelkirk, Janet L. & Fody, Edward P. (2000). *Clinical Chemistry: Principles, Procedures Correlations.* 4th ed. Philadelphia: J. B. Lippincott.

Burtis, Carl A. & Ashwood, Edward R. (1999). *Tietz Textbook of Clinical Chemistry.* 3rd ed. Philadelphia: W. B. Saunders.

Burtis, Carl A. & Ashwood, Edward R. (2001). *Tietz Fundamentals of Clinical Chemistry.* 5th ed. Philadelphia: W. B. Saunders.

Kleinschmidt, Paul. (2000). *Chronic Obstructive Pulmonary Disease and Emphysema.* [On-line] Available: www.emedicine.com/emerg/topic99.htm [2000, September 5].

Lehman, Craig A. (1998). *Saunders Manual of Clinical Laboratory Science.* Philadelphia: W. B. Saunders.

CHEMISTRY CASE 2–9

Joe M., a 52-year-old man, came to the ER with an extremely inflamed big toe, chills, and fever. He had recently attended a niece's wedding, where he had eaten a lot of rich food and imbibed a larger amount of alcohol than normal. His physician ordered the laboratory tests shown in Tables 2–19 to 2–21.

■ Table 2–19 ■   CHEMISTRY PANEL

	Joe M.	Reference Range
Sodium	139	136–145 mEq/L
Potassium	4.2	3.6–5.0 mEq/L
Chloride	104	101–111 mEq/L
CO_2	27.0	24.0–34.0 mEq/L
Glucose	100	80–120 mg/dL
Bilirubin, total	0.3	0.2–1.2 mg/dL
AST	25	5–40 IU/L
ALP	42	30–157 IU/L
Total protein	6.5	6.0–8.4 g/dL
BUN	20	7–24 mg/dL
Creatinine	0.9	0.5–1.2 mg/dL
Calcium	8.8	8.5–10.5 mg/dL
Uric acid	11.5	3.5–5.2 mg/dL
Albumin	3.6	3.5–5.0 g/dL

■ Table 2–20 ■   HEMATOLOGY RESULTS

	Joe M..	Reference Range
CBC		
WBC	15.0	$5–10 \times 10^9$/L
RBC	5.04	$5–6 \times 10^{12}$/L
Hb	153	135–175 g/L
Hct	.46	.41–.53 L/L
MCV	92	80–100 fL
MCH	29	26–34 pg
MCHC	33	31–37%
Platelets	240	$150–400 \times 10^9$/L
Segs	64	25–60%
Band	0	0–10%
Lymphocytes	21	20–50%
Monocytes	14	2–11%
Eosinophils	0	0–8%

■ Table 2–20 ■   HEMATOLOGY RESULTS *(continued)*

	Joe M.	Reference Range
CBC		
Basophils	1	0–2%
Atypical lymphocytes	0	0–5%
RBC morphology	Normal	Normal
ESR	30 mm/h	(0–15 mm/h)

■ Table 2–21 ■   URINALYSIS

	Joe M.	Reference Range
Macroscopic		
Color	Yellow	Colorless to amber
Appearance	Clear	Clear
Specific gravity	1.022	1.001–1.035
pH	6.0	5–7
Protein	Neg	Neg
Glucose	Neg	Neg
Ketones	Neg	Neg
Bilirubin	Neg	Neg
Blood	Neg	Neg
Urobilinogen	Normal	Normal
Nitrite	Neg	Neg
Leukocyte esterase	Neg	Neg
Microscopic		
WBCs	0–2/HPF	0–5/HPF
RBCs	0–1/HPF	0–2/HPF
Epithelial cells	Rare squamous/HPF	Few to moderate
Casts	0–1 hyaline/LPF	Few hyaline
Crystals	Many uric acid	

QUESTIONS

1. List or highlight the abnormal laboratory results.

2. Based on the laboratory results and medical history, what is the most probable diagnosis?

3.   a. What are the two main types of hyperuricemia (increased uric acid)?

   b. List five conditions under each category.

4. List at least four risk factors for the development of this condition.

5. What is the epidemiology of this condition? (What demographic groups are associated with this condition?)

6. What is the pathophysiology of this condition; in other words, what happens in the body?

7. If Joe's physician performed an arthrocentesis (puncture of a joint space with a needle to aspirate accumulated fluid), what would you expect to find in the joint fluid?

8. What types of food should Joe avoid? List six foods that should *not* be part of his daily diet.

9. What three renal complications are associated with this condition?

10. Briefly discuss two medications used to treat this condition and how they work (medications used to treat the disease, *not* the symptoms, but the underlying problem—to prevent recurrent attacks).

RECOMMENDED READINGS

Bishop, Michael L., Duben-Engelkirk, Janet L. & Fody, Edward P. (2000). *Clinical Chemistry: Principles, Procedures Correlations.* 4th ed. Philadelphia: J. B. Lippincott.

Burtis, Carl A. & Ashwood, Edward R. (1999). *Tietz Textbook of Clinical Chemistry.* 3rd ed. Philadelphia: W. B. Saunders.

Burtis, Carl A. & Ashwood, Edward R. (2001). *Tietz Fundamentals of Clinical Chemistry.* 5th ed. Philadelphia: W. B. Saunders.

Pittman, Joel R. & Bross, Michael H. (1999). *Diagnosis and Management of Gout.* [Online] Available: www.aafp.org/afp/990401ap/1799.html [2000, September 5].

CHEMISTRY CASE 2–10

Mike L., a 47-year-old man, went to his physician for an "annual" physical that had been postponed for over 3 years. He had started his own business 4 years ago and had been extremely busy getting it established. Mike's medical history indicated he was a nonsmoker, and his father and grandfather had histories of myocardial infarctions before age 55. Since she had not seen this patient in a number of years, the physician decided to order routine screening tests. See Tables 2–22 and 2–23.

■ Table 2–22 ■ CHEMISTRY RESULTS

	Mike L.	Reference Range
Sodium	143	136–145 mEq/L
Potassium	4.6	3.6–5.0 mEq/L
Chloride	104	101–111 mEq/L
CO_2	29.0	24.0–34.0 mEq/L
Glucose	95	80–120 mg/dL
BUN	19	7–24 mg/dL
Creatinine	1.0	0.5–1.2 mg/dL
Bilirubin, total	0.5	0.2–1.2 mg/dL
AST	35	5–40 IU/L
ALP	70	30–157 IU/L
Total protein	7.5	6.0–8.4 g/dL
Albumin	4.6	3.5–5.0 g/dL
Calcium	8.5	8.5–10.5 mg/dL

Miscellaneous Chemistry

Cholesterol	305	Recommended (desirable): <200 mg/dL

■ Table 2–23 ■ URINALYSIS

	Mike L.	Reference Range
Macroscopic		
Color	Yellow	Colorless to amber
Appearance	Clear	Clear
Specific gravity	1.014	1.001–1.035
pH	6.0	5–7
Protein	Neg	Neg
Glucose	Neg	Neg
Ketones	Neg	Neg
Bilirubin	Neg	Neg
Blood	Neg	Neg
Urobilinogen	Normal	Normal

■ Table 2–23 ■ URINALYSIS (continued)

	Mike L.	Reference Range
Macroscopic		
Nitrite	Neg	Neg
Leukocyte esterase	Neg	Neg
Microscopic		
Not Indicated		

QUESTIONS

1. Circle or highlight the abnormal result(s) in Table 2–22 and 2–23.

2. List at least eight secondary conditions/disorders associated with the abnormal result(s) in question 1.

3. Which of the conditions you listed for question 2 can the physician rule out with Mike's medical history, physical examination, and current laboratory results?

4. What is the most probable cause of the abnormal result in this patient?

The following week, a lipid profile was performed on a 12-hour fasting specimen (Table 2–24).

■ **Table 2–24** ■ **LIPID PROFILE**

	Mike L.	Reference Range
Cholesterol	305	Recommended (desirable): < 200 mg/dL
HDL cholesterol	45	29–75 mg/dL
Triglycerides	390	Recommended (desirable): < 250 mg/dL

5. Given the above information, what is Mike's LDL cholesterol (LDLC)? Based on his LDLC, is he at high risk for coronary heart disease (CHD), moderate risk, or within the recommended (desirable) range?

6. a. If Mike's triglycerides were 450 mg/dL, could the LDLC be calculated? Why or why not?

   b. What would be the next step?

7. List eight risk factors associated with CHD as determined by the National Cholesterol Education Program (NCEP) Adult Treatment Panel.

8. How many risk factors does Mike presently have, given the information provided? Is he at high risk for CHD?

9. What are the follow-up testing and treatment recommendations by the NCEP Adult Treatment Panel?

10. List at least three types of drugs used to treat this condition and their effect (how they work and what they lower or decrease).

RECOMMENDED READINGS

Bishop, Michael L., Duben-Engelkirk, Janet L. & Fody, Edward P. (2000). *Clinical Chemistry: Principles, Procedures Correlations*. 4th ed. Philadelphia: J. B. Lippincott.

Burtis, Carl A. & Ashwood, Edward R. (1999). *Tietz Textbook of Clinical Chemistry*. 3rd ed. Philadelphia: W. B. Saunders.

Burtis, Carl A. & Ashwood, Edward R. (2001). *Tietz Fundamentals of Clinical Chemistry*. 5th ed. Philadelphia: W. B. Saunders.

Lehman, Craig A. (1998). *Saunders Manual of Clinical Laboratory Science*. Philadelphia: W. B. Saunders.

National Cholesterol Education Program (NCEP). (1993). *Second Report of the Expert Panel on Detection, Evaluation, and Treatment of High Cholesterol in Adults (Adult Treatment Panel II)*. [On-line] Available: www.nhlbi.nih.gov/guidelines/-choleseterol/atp_sum.htm [2000, November 6].

CHEMISTRY CASE 2–11

Marie H., a 42-year-old woman, was admitted to the ER with complaints of nausea, vomiting, chills, fever, and severe right upper quadrant pain. She had experienced similar symptoms a "few" times in the last 6 months, but the episodes had been much milder and had disappeared in 2 or 3 hours. The ER physician noted she was visibly jaundiced. See Tables 2–25 to 2–28.

■ Table 2–25 ■   LIVER PROFILE

	Marie H.	Reference Range
Bilirubin, total	15.5	0.2–1.2 mg/dL
Bilirubin, direct	10.3	0.00–0.40 mg/dL
AST	100	5–40 IU/L
ALP	645	30–157 IU/L
ALT	105	5–40 IU/L
Albumin	4.0	3.5–5.0 g/dL
Total protein	7.4	6.0–8.4 g/dL
γGT	400	2–30 IU/L

■ Table 2–26 ■   CHEMISTRY TESTS

Amylase	120	27–131 U/L
Cholesterol	330	Recommended (desirable): < 200 mg/dL
Triglycerides	238	Recommended (desirable): < 250 mg/dL

■ Table 2–27 ■   Complete Blood Count

	Marie H.	Reference Range
WBC	15.4	$5–10 \times 10^9$/L
RBC	5.10	$4.0–5.0 \times 10^{12}$/L
Hb	146	120–160 g/L
Hct	.44	.36–.46 L/L
MCV	97	80–100 fL
MCH	30	26–34 pg
MCHC	35	31–37%
Platelets	250	$150–400 \times 10^9$/L
Segmented neutrophils	75	25–60%
Lymphocytes	15	20–50%
Monocytes	7	2–11%
Eosinophils	3	0–8%
Basophils	0	0–2%
RBC morphology	Normal	Normal

■ **Table 2–28** ■ URINALYSIS

	Marie H.	Reference Range
Macroscopic		
Color	Dark amber	Colorless to amber
Appearance	Clear	Clear
Specific gravity	1.013	1.001–1.035
pH	6.0	5–7
Protein	Neg	Neg
Glucose	Neg	Neg
Ketones	Neg	Neg
Bilirubin	2+	Neg
Blood	Neg	Neg
Urobilinogen	Normal	Normal
Nitrite	Neg	Neg
Leukocyte esterase	Neg	Neg
Microscopic		
WBCs	0–2/HPF	0–5/HPF
RBCs	0–1/HPF	0–2/HPF
Epithelial cells	Few squamous/HPF	Few to moderate
Casts	0–2 hyaline/LPF	Few hyaline
Bacteria	Neg	None

QUESTIONS

1. Circle or highlight the abnormal results.

2. List five conditions that could produce these physical symptoms that the physician should rule in or out.

3. What is the most likely explanation for Marie's pain?

4. Do the laboratory data support your explanation in question 3?

5. Can the physician rule out any of the conditions you listed in question 2? How, what tests?

6.   a. What is the chemical composition of the stones associated with this condition?

      b. How are they formed?

7. List four risk factors for this condition.

8. Would the color of Marie's stools be described as normal (brown)? If not, what color would this be and why?

9. Is Marie's urine urobilinogen in fact "normal"? If not, why?

RECOMMENDED READINGS

Bishop, Michael L., Duben-Engelkirk, Janet L. & Fody, Edward P. (2000). *Clinical Chemistry: Principles, Procedures Correlations.* 4th ed. Philadelphia: J. B. Lippincott.

Burtis, Carl A. & Ashwood, Edward R. (1999). *Tietz Textbook of Clinical Chemistry.* 3rd ed. Philadelphia: W. B. Saunders.

Burtis, Carl A. & Ashwood, Edward R. (2001). *Tietz Fundamentals of Clinical Chemistry.* 5th ed. Philadelphia: W. B. Saunders.

Damjanov, Ivan. (1996). *Pathology for the Health-Related Professions.* Philadelphia: W. B. Saunders.

Santen, Sally. (2000). *Cholecystitis and Biliary Colic.* [On-line] Available: www.emedicine.com/topic98.htm [2000, September 5].

CHEMISTRY CASE 2–12

James T., a 55-year-old man, visited his physician because he noticed abdominal swelling and complained of fatigue and weakness. Upon physical examination, the physician noted icteric (jaundiced) sclera (outer layer of the eyeball, e.g., white of the eyes), some edema around the ankles, splenomegaly, and hepatomegaly. James also admitted to drinking at least five martinis every night and more on weekends for a number of years. The tests in Tables 2–29 to 2–31 were ordered.

■ Table 2–29 ■ CHEMISTRY TESTS/ LIVER PROFILE

	James T.	Reference Range
Bilirubin, total	2.5	0.2–1.2 mg/dL
Bilirubin, direct	1.51	0.00–0.40 mg/dL
AST	350	5–40 IU/L
ALP	214	30–157 IU/L
ALT	200	5–40 IU/L
Albumin	3.0	3.5–5.0 g/dL
γGT	300	2–30 IU/L
Total protein	7.2	6.0–8.4 g/dL
Cholesterol	160	Recommended (desirable): < 200 mg/dL

■ Table 2–30 ■ HEMATOLOGY

	James T.	Reference Range
CBC		
WBC	6.0	$4.8–10.8 \times 10^9$/L
RBC	4.80	$4.70–6.10 \times 10^{12}$/L
Hb	155	140–180 g/L
Hct	.49	.41–.53 L/L
MCV	102	80–100 fL
MCH	32	26–34 pg
MCHC	32	31–37%
Platelets	150	$150–400 \times 10^9$/L
Segs	65	25–60%
Lymphocytes	20	20–50%
Monocytes	10	2–11%
Eosinophils	4	0–8%
Basophils	1	0–2%
RBC morphology	Normal	Normal
Prothrombin time	16	12–14 seconds

■ Table 2–31 ■ HEPATITIS SERUM PANEL

	James T.	Reference Range
Anti-HCV	Nonreactive	Nonreactive
Anti-HAV (IgM)	Nonreactive	Nonreactive
Anti-HAV (total)	Nonreactive	Nonreactive
Anti-HBsAg	Nonreactive	Nonreactive
Anti-HBcAg	Nonreactive	Nonreactive

QUESTIONS

1. Circle or highlight the abnormal results in Tables 2–29 and 2–30.

2. What organ is involved?

3. Briefly describe the pathophysiology (the pathological changes) in the organ in this condition.

4. List five etiologies (causes) of this condition.

5. Given the results of James's physical examination, history, and laboratory tests, what etiology is the most probable cause of this disease?

6. Explain why the prothrombin time is prolonged and the albumin decreased.

7. What is the cause of the macrocytosis?

8.   a. What is the cause of the abdominal swelling?

   b. What symptoms associated with this condition result in abdominal swelling?

9. List and briefly describe three complications associated with this condition.

10. What test would the physician order if he or she suspected impending hepatic coma?

RECOMMENDED READINGS

Bishop, Michael L., Duben-Engelkirk, Janet L. & Fody, Edward P. (2000). *Clinical Chemistry: Principles, Procedures Correlations*. 4th ed. Philadelphia: J. B. Lippincott.

Burtis, Carl A. & Ashwood, Edward R. (1999). *Tietz Textbook of Clinical Chemistry*. 3rd ed. Philadelphia: W. B. Saunders.

Burtis, Carl A. & Ashwood, Edward R. (2001). *Tietz Fundamentals of Clinical Chemistry*. 5th ed. Philadelphia: W. B. Saunders.

Kaplan, Lawrence A. & Pesce, Amadeo J. (1996). *Clinical Chemistry: Theory, Analysis, Correlation*. 3rd ed. St. Louis: Mosby.

Lehman, Craig A. (1998). *Saunders Manual of Clinical Laboratory Science*. Philadelphia: W. B. Saunders.

Hematology

Kathryn Doig, Ph.D.

HEMATOLOGY CASE 3–1

A complete blood count (CBC), reticulocyte count, and bilirubin were ordered on a 2-hour-old white newborn male, Baby Boy C. The laboratory results are shown in Tables 3–1 and 3–2.

■ Table 3–1 ■ CBC AND RETICULOCYTE COUNT

	Baby Boy C.	Newborn Reference Ranges or Mean Values*	Early Childhood Reference Ranges or Mean Values*	Adult Male Reference Range*
WBC count ($\times 10^9$/L)	17.3	9–30	5.5–15.5	5–10
RBC count ($\times 10^{12}$/L)	4.07	3.9–5.5	3.9–5.3	5–6
Hb (g/L)	135	145–205	115–135	135–175
Hct (L/L)	.41	.42–.60	.34–.40	.41–.53
MCV (fL)	102	98–118	75–87	80–100
MCH (g/dL)	31.6	31–37	24–30	26–34
MCHC (%)	32.5	30–36	31–37	31–37
RDW-CV (%)	16.5	15–19[†]	12–14[†]	11.5–14.5
Platelets ($\times 10^9$/L)	223	192		150–400
Differential (%)				
Neutrophils	51	61[‡]	41[§]	25–60
Bands	2			0–10
Lymphocytes	41	31	50	20–50
Monocytes	6	6	5	2–11
Eosinophils	0	2	3	0–8
Basophils	0	0	0	0–2
Morphology	2+ anisocytosis, 2+ poikilocytosis, 2+ macrocytes, 1+ spherocytes, 3+ polychromasia, 13 NRBC/100 WBC			
Reticulocytes (%)	11	3–7		0.5–2

*Handin, Lux, & Stossel, 1995.
[†]Auerbach & Alter, 1989.
[‡]Includes bands that may constitute as much as 50% of the granulocytes.
[§]Includes bands that may constitute as much as 30% of the granulocytes.
Abbreviations: CBC, complete blood count; Hb, hemoglobin; Hct, hematocrit; MCH, mean corpuscular hemoglobin; MCHC, mean corpuscular hemoglobin concentration; MCV, mean corpuscular volume; NRBC, nucleated red blood cell; RBC, red blood cell; RDW-CV, red blood cell distribution width index—coefficient of variation; WBC, white blood cell.

■ Table 3–2 ■   BILIRUBIN RESULTS

	Baby Boy C.	Reference Range
Total bilirubin	4.2	0.2–1.2 mg/dL
Direct bilirubin	0.3	0.1–0.3 mg/dL

QUESTIONS

1. The quantitative parameters reported in the CBC in Table 3–1 are taken directly from the instrument.

   a. Are they reportable?

   b. If not, why not, and what must be done before the results can be reported?

   c. How is this done?

2. With a corrected WBC count, Baby Boy C.'s WBCs can be evaluated. Are any abnormalities noted?

3. . a. Why is the reference range of the WBC count for newborns higher than for adults?

Stressful birth
marginating neutrophils

b. Why is the percentage of neutrophils higher in newborns than in older children, and why is the percentage of lymphocytes higher in children than in adults?

4. a. Is this baby anemic?

b. If so, describe the anemia using Wintrobe's morphological descriptions.

5. a. Would an adult with comparable RBC values be considered anemic?

        b. Why do infants have higher reference values for judging anemia?

6.   a. Interpret the morphological appearance of the RBCs, including correlation with the measured parameters.

        b. Does the morphological description of the RBCs offer any clues to the cause of the anemia?

7. What other findings are consistent with the possibility of an extravascular hemolytic process?

8.   a. Is the reticulocyte response sufficient to correct the baby's anemia within a reasonable length of time if the cause of hemolysis is removed?

b. How will you decide?

9.   a. How can the absolute number of reticulocytes be determined?

b. What advantage does this provide?

10.   a. In a newborn demonstrating evidence of a hemolytic anemia, what is the most likely cause?

b. What other condition may produce similar findings in a newborn?

11. Can the hematology results provide clues to the blood group causing the hemolytic disease of the newborn (HDN)?

REFERENCES

Auerbach, A. D. & Alter, B. P. (1989). Prenatal and postnatal diagnosis of aplastic anemia. In Alter, B. P. (Ed.), *Perinatal Hematology*. London: Churchill Livingstone.

Handin, R. I., Lux, S. E. & Stossel, T. P. (Eds.). (1995). *Blood: Principles and Practice of Hematology*. Philadelphia: J. B. Lippincott.

RECOMMENDED READINGS

Clark, K. & Hippel, C. (2000). Routine testing in hematology. In Rodak, B. *Hematology: Clinical Principles and Applications*. 2nd ed. Philadelphia: W. B. Saunders.

McKenzie, S. B. (1996a). The erythrocyte. In McKenzie, S. B. (Ed.), *Textbook of Hematology*. 2nd ed. Baltimore: Williams & Wilkins.

McKenzie, S. B. (1996b). Myeloproliferative disorders. In McKenzie, S. B. (Ed.), *Textbook of Hematology*. 2nd ed. Baltimore: Williams & Wilkins.

Tonte, A. & Stevens, A. (1995). Pediatric and geriatric hematology. In Rodak, B. F. (Ed.), *Diagnostic Hematology*. Philadelphia: W. B. Saunders.

HEMATOLOGY CASE 3–2

Fred G., a 22-year-old white man, was seen in the emergency department of a small rural hospital following a motorcycle crash. He was disoriented and in shock at the time of admission, and although he had bruises and contusions, he did not appear to be bleeding externally. The physician ordered a stat urinalysis, CBC, and type and hold for 2 Units of packed red blood cells. The blood samples were drawn from the patient's right wrist while a nurse attempted to insert an intravenous (IV) line in the other arm. Both procedures were difficult to achieve. See Table 3–3.

■ **Table 3–3** ■ **COMPLETE BLOOD COUNT**

	Fred G.	Adult Male Reference Range*
WBC count	16.5	$5–10 \times 10^9$/L
RBC count	4.77	$5–6 \times 10^{12}$/L
Hb	143	135–175 g/L
Hct	.43	.41–.53 L/L
MCV	85	80–100 fL
MCH	30	26–34 pg
MCHC	33	31–37 g/dL
RDW-CV	12	11.5–14.5%
Platelets	439	$150–400 \times 10^9$/L
Differential		
Neutrophils	83	25–60%
Bands	2	0–10%
Lymphocytes	15	20–50%
Monocytes	0	2–11%
Eosinophils	0	0–8%
Basophils	0	0–2%
Morphology	Unremarkable	

*Handin, Lux, & Stossel, 1995.

QUESTIONS

1. Explain any patient values outside the reference range in light of the history provided.

The physician ordered a repeat hemoglobin (Hb) and hematocrit (Hct) on the patient, 45 minutes later. At this time, the Hb was 118 g/L and the Hct was .35 L/L. In the meantime, a catheterized urinalysis sample was received in the laboratory. The sample was grossly bloody, approaching the appearance of whole blood.

2.   a. Provide two explanations for the drop of nearly 30 g/L of Hb over the 45-minute time frame.

      b. Predict the relative effect (increase, decrease, or unchanged) on the WBC count and platelet count.

3.   a. Which Hb measurement is the best representation of the patient's actual level of Hb: the one collected at admission to the emergency department or the one collected 45 minutes later?

      b. Explain your choice.

4.   a. Explain why the size and shape of the RBCs remain normal despite the development of anemia in a patient with acute hemorrhage.

     b. Distinguish this from the RBC appearance in chronic hemorrhage, and explain the difference.

5.   a. What morphological change would you expect to this patient's peripheral blood smear over the next week, and what does it represent?

     b. What is the physiologic mechanism mediating this response?

     c. How would this be affected if the patient is transfused with RBCs?

6. a. Distinguish relative erythrocytosis from absolute erythrocytosis.

    b. Distinguish primary erythrocytosis from secondary erythrocytosis, including erythropoietin levels.

    c. Provide examples of each.

    d. Which are considered appropriate and which are inappropriate physiological responses?

REFERENCES

Handin, R. I., Lux, S. E. & Stossel, T. P. (Eds.). (1995). *Blood: Principles and Practice of Hematology*. Philadelphia: J. B. Lippincott.

RECOMMENDED READINGS

Bullock, B. L. (1996). Shock. In Bullock, B. L. (Ed.), *Pathophysiology: Adaptations and Alternations in Function*. 4th ed. Philadelphia: J. B. Lippincott.

Clark, K. & Hippel, T. G. (1995). Miscellaneous erythrocyte disorders. In Rodak, B. F. (Ed.), *Diagnostic Hematology*. Philadelphia: W. B. Saunders.

McKenzie, S. B. (1996). Myeloproliferative disorders. In McKenzie, S. B. (Ed.), *Textbook of Hematology*. 2nd ed. Baltimore: Williams & Wilkins.

HEMATOLOGY CASE 3–3

Jean L., a 30-year-old white woman, was seen in the office of a rheumatologist. She was diagnosed in childhood with rheumatoid arthritis. Even at the relatively young age of 30 years, the joints of her hands were noticeably enlarged and deformed, and her gait was affected by knee and hip pain. See Table 3–4.

■ Table 3–4 ■ COMPLETE BLOOD COUNT

	Jean L.	Adult Female Reference Range*
WBC count	12.1	$5–10 \times 10^9$/L
RBC count	4.23	$4.0–15.0 \times 10^{12}$/L
Hb	105	120–160 g/L
Hct	.33	.36–.46 L/L
MCV	78	80–100 fL
MCH	25	26–34 pg
MCHC	32	31–37 g/dL
RDW-CV	15	11.5–14.5%
Platelets	230	$150–400 \times 10^9$/L
Differential		
Neutrophils	45	25–60%
Bands	2	0–10%
Lymphocytes	46	20–50%
Monocytes	7	2–11%
Eosinophils	0	0–8%
Basophils	0	0–2%
Morphology	Unremarkable	

*Handin, Lux, & Stossel, 1995.

QUESTIONS

1. Based on the CBC results presented, describe Jean's blood picture, including WBCs, RBCs, and platelets.

2.   a. Name three causes of anemia that produce RBCs with an MCV like Jean's.

      b. Briefly describe the pathogenesis of each of these anemias.

3. Considering the patient's gender, age, and medical history, which two conditions are more likely to account for Jean's RBC picture?

4. How can the RDW be used to assist in the differential diagnosis of Jean's condition?

5.   a. What tests can be used to distinguish the diseases in question 2?

b. What results are expected in each condition and why?

6. Describe the principle and any calculations involved for measuring serum iron, iron-binding capacity, percent saturation, ferritin, zinc protopor-phyrin, and serum transferrin receptors.

The physician ordered iron studies for this patient, including ferritin (see Table 3–5).

■ Table 3–5 ■ IRON STUDIES

	Jean L.	Reference Range
Total serum iron	45	40–180 µg/dL
Total iron-binding capacity	320	250–420 µg/dL
% Saturation	14	15–50%
Ferritin	80	10–300 µg/L

7. The physician was skeptical that the ferritin result accurately represented the patient's iron status. Why?

8. To avoid the invasiveness of a bone marrow sample, what other test could be helpful in determining whether this patient is iron deficient?

REFERENCES

Handin, R. I., Lux, S. E. & Stossel, T. P. (Eds.), (1995). *Blood: Principles and Practice of Hematology*. Philadelphia: J. B. Lippincott.

RECOMMENDED READINGS

Doig, K. (2000). Disorders of iron metabolism. In Rodak, B. F. (Ed.), *Hematology: Clinical Principles and Applications*. Philadelphia: W. B. Saunders.

McKenzie, S. B. (1996). Anemia of defective heme synthesis. In McKenzie, S. B. (Ed.), *Textbook of Hematology*. 2nd ed. Baltimore: Williams & Wilkins.

HEMATOLOGY CASE 3–4

Ryan L., a 6-year-old white boy, was seen by a maxillofacial surgeon to be evaluated for surgical repair of severe jaw misalignment. The youngster was deemed an appropriate candidate for surgery at this time, with a second surgery planned during his teen years to complete the correction. The child was adopted, and no family history was available. He had no personal history of excessive bleeding or bruising. The presurgical CBC results including platelet count were within reference ranges. Presurgical hemostasis testing follows:

	Ryan L.	Reference Range
Prothrombin time	10.5	9–12 s
APTT	40	32–46 s
Bleeding time	7	1–9 min

Abbreviations: APTT, activated partial thromboplastin time; s, seconds.

QUESTIONS

1. Describe the principle and reagents for the APTT and prothrombin time.

Ryan was taken to surgery but experienced excessive bleeding during surgery and continued oozing and bleeding postoperatively. Prothrombin time, APTT, and bleeding times performed postoperatively follow:

	Ryan L.	Reference Range
Prothrombin time	10.5	9–12 s
APTT	48	32–46 s
Bleeding time	8	1–9 min

2. Assuming that the patient has a hemostatic system abnormality,
   a. Can the cause be narrowed by the results of the preceding screening tests?

b. If yes, to what factor(s) of the hemostatic system is(are) the abnor-mality(ies) confined?

3. What additional testing is indicated to identify the cause of Ryan's contin-ued bleeding, and what is the principle of this test?

4. How is "correction" of a mixing study determined, and why is it needed?

Results of prothrombin time and APTT using a 1:1 mix of patient and reagent normal plasma gave the following results:

	Ryan L.	Reference Range
Prothrombin time	11	9–12 s
Reagent normal plasma PT	10	
APTT	40	32–46 s
Reagent normal plasma APTT	36	

Abbreviation: PT, prothrombin time

5. Interpret the results of the 1:1 mixing studies to narrow the patient's abnor-mality further.

6.   a. What testing can be done to further narrow the possible factor deficiencies?

b. Describe how the test is performed and the results expected for various factor deficiencies.

7. Factor-deficient plasmas are expensive, so testing should be done in a logical fashion based on the factors most likely to be deficient. For which factors and in what order should this patient be tested? Justify your decision.

Factor Assay Results

Factor VIII	75% of normal
Factor IX	3% of normal

8.   a. What factor is apparently affected in this patient?

     b. What is the condition called?

9. Compare this condition to hemophilia A, including

     a. Deficient factor

     b. Pattern of inheritance

     c. Gender affected

d. Clinical presentation

e. Incidence

f. Incidence among hereditary coagulation factor deficiencies

g. Treatment

10.   a. What is the general reference range for percent of normal for coagu-
         lation factors?

b. What is the level of mild versus severe deficiencies in hemophilia?

11. How could an individual have a normal amount of a coagulation factor but still have a prolonged screening test or deficient factor assay result?

12. What is the difference in clinical presentation between individuals with a factor deficiency and those with a defective molecule of the same factor?

13. a. How do hereditary factor deficiencies differ from acquired deficiencies?

b. List examples of acquired coagulation factor deficiencies.

c. Which are more common: hereditary or acquired deficiencies?

RECOMMENDED READINGS

Fritsma G. (2000a). Evaluation of hemostasis. In Rodak B. F. (Ed.), *Hematology: Clinical Principles and Applications*. Philadelphia: W. B. Saunders.

Fritsma, G. (2000b). Hemorrhagic coagulation disorders. In Rodak B. F. (Ed.), *Hematology: Clinical Principles and Applications*. Philadelphia: W. B. Saunders.

Fritsma G. (2000c). Normal hemostasis and coagulation. In Rodak B. F. (Ed.), *Hematology: Clinical Principles and Applications*. Philadelphia: W. B. Saunders.

Larson, L. (1996a). Disorders of secondary hemostasis. In MacKenzie S. B. (Ed.), *Textbook of Hematology*. 2nd ed. Baltimore: Williams & Wilkins.

Larson, L. (1996b). Laboratory methods in coagulation. In MacKenzie S. B. (Ed.), *Textbook of Hematology*. 2nd ed. Baltimore: Williams & Wilkins.

HEMATOLOGY CASE 3–5

Ellen P., a 35-year-old white woman, had a history of systemic lupus erythematosus, diagnosed when she was in her early twenties. Her disease was generally under good control with steroid treatments. However, she was admitted to the hospital due to a recent onset of jaundice. Her liver was enlarged and tender.

Among her admission laboratory results are those shown in Table 3–6.

■ Table 3–6 ■   COMPLETE BLOOD COUNT

	Ellen P.	Adult Female Reference Range[*]	Reference Range for Absolute Values ($\times 10^9$/L)
WBC count	13.5	$5–10 \times 10^9$/L	
RBC count	3.63	$4.0–5.0 \times 10^{12}$/L	
Hb	109	120–160 g/L	
Hct	.33	.36–.46 L/L	
MCV	91	80–100 fL	
MCH	30	26–34 pg	
MCHC	33	31–37 g/dL	
RDW-CV	12	11.5–14.5%	
Platelets	139	$150–400 \times 10^9$/L	
Differential			
Neutrophils	43	25–60%	1.10–6.05
Bands	0	0–10%	0.10–2.1
Lymphocytes	55	20–50%	1.50–4.00
Monocytes	2	2–11%	0.20–0.95
Eosinophils	0	0–8%	0–0.70
Basophils	0	0–2%	0–0.15
Morphology	50% of lymphocytes are reactive		

[*]Handin, Lux, & Stossel, 1995.

QUESTIONS

1. a. Describe Ellen's blood picture using appropriate terminology.

b. Determine whether any elevations or decreases among WBCs are relative and/or absolute.

2. What conditions produce a blood picture like Ellen's, and which is most likely in her case?

3. Explain the etiology of the lymphocyte appearance.

Tests for liver enzymes were elevated, and acute hepatitis C was diagnosed. While in the hospital, Ellen developed pain, swelling, and redness in the left calf, attributable to a venous thrombus. See Table 3–7.

■ Table 3–7 ■   SCREENING COAGULATION TEST RESULTS

	Ellen P.	Reference Range
Prothrombin time	10	9–13 s
APTT	42	28–34 s

4.   a. What might explain a prolonged APTT from a patient apparently experiencing a thrombotic event?

b. Why does this occur?

5. Describe screening and confirmatory testing for antiphospholipid antibodies.

6. What other laboratory tests may be affected by the presence of antiphospholipid antibodies?

REFERENCES

Handin, R. I., Lux, S. E. & Stossel, T. P. (Eds.). (1995). *Blood: Principles and Practice of Hematology*. Philadelphia: J. B. Lippincott.

RECOMMENDED READINGS

Fritsma, G. (2000a). Evaluation of hemostasis. In Rodak, B. F. (Ed.), *Hematology: Clinical Principles and Applications*. Philadelphia: W. B. Saunders.

Fritsma, G. (2000b). Normal hemostasis and coagulation. In Rodak, B. F. (Ed.) *Hematology: Clinical Principles and Applications*. Philadelphia: W. B. Saunders.

Fritsma, G. (2000c). Thrombotic risk testing. In Rodak, B. F. (Ed.), *Hematology: Clinical Principles and Applications*. Philadelphia: W. B. Saunders.

Larson, L. (1996). Disorders of secondary hemostasis. In MacKenzie S. B. (Ed.), *Textbook of Hematology*. 2nd ed. Baltimore: Williams & Wilkins.

Leclair, S. (2000). Leukopoiesis. In Rodak, B. F. (Ed.), *Hematology: Clinical Principles and Applications*. Philadelphia: W. B. Saunders.

McKenzie, S. B. (1996). Nonmalignant lymphocyte disorders. In McKenzie, S. B. (Ed.), *Textbook of Hematology*. 2nd ed. Baltimore: Williams & Wilkins.

HEMATOLOGY CASE 3–6

Geoff J., a 54-year-old white man, was seen in the emergency department of a large metropolitan hospital. The man was homeless and alcoholic. He was brought to the hospital by the director of a homeless shelter. The director was concerned about allowing the man to stay at the shelter because he appeared seriously ill and might be infectious to others. Geoff was experiencing fever, chills, and a deep productive cough. See Table 3–8.

■ Table 3–8 ■   COMPLETE BLOOD COUNT

	Geoff J.	Adult Male Reference Range*	Reference Range for Absolute Values ($\times 10^9$/L)
WBC count	18.3	5–10×10^9/L	
RBC count	3.1	5–6×10^{12}/L	
Hb	110	135–175 g/L	
Hct	.34	.41–.53 L/L	
MCV	108	80–100 fL	
MCH	35	26–34 pg	
MCHC	34	31–37 g/dL	
RDW-CV	16	11.5–14.5%	
Platelets	237	150–400×10^9/L	
Differential (%)			
Neutrophils	75	25–60%	1.10–6.05
Bands	15	0–10%	0.10–2.1
Lymphocytes	10	20–50%	1.50–4.00
Monocytes	0	2–11%	0.20–0.95
Eosinophils	0	0–8%	0–0.70
Basophils	0	0–2%	0–0.15
Morphology	1+ macrocytosis, occ. target cell, toxic granulation, vacuolization, occ. Döhle bodies		

*Handin, Lux, & Stossel, 1995.

QUESTIONS

1.   a. Describe Geoff's blood picture using appropriate terminology.

b. Determine whether any elevations or decreases among WBCs are relative and/or absolute.

2. Explain the etiology of the WBC abnormalities noted using appropriate terminology.

3. For Geoff, what is the likely explanation for the WBC abnormalities described in Table 3–8?

4.   a. Describe the RBC parameters for Geoff and their likely etiology.

      b. Discuss the mechanism by which anemia develops in this condition.

5. The RBC morphology described for Geoff can be seen in other conditions. What conditions are those, and how would the anemia of alcoholism be differentiated from those conditions?

REFERENCES

Handin, R. I., Lux, S. E. & Stossel, T. P. (Eds.) (1995). *Blood: Principles and Practice of Hematology*. Philadelphia: J. B. Lippincott.

RECOMMENDED READINGS

Bradford, C. (2000). Cytochemistry. In Rodak, B. F. (Ed.), *Hematology: Clinical Principles and Applications*. Philadelphia: W. B. Saunders.

Leclair, S. (2000). Qualitative leukocyte disorders. In Rodak, B. F. (Ed.), *Hematology: Clinical Principles and Applications*. Philadelphia: W. B. Saunders.

Leclair, S. (2000). Quantitative leukocyte disorders. In Rodak, B. F. (Ed.), *Hematology: Clinical Principles and Applications*. Philadelphia: W. B. Saunders.

McKenzie, S. J. (1996). Nonmalignant granulocyte and monocyte disorders. In McKenzie, S. B. (Ed.), *Textbook of Hematology*. 2nd ed. Baltimore: Williams & Wilkins.

HEMATOLOGY CASE 3–7

Thomas H., a 5-year-old African American boy, was seen in the office of his primary care physician. His mother had insisted on an immediate appointment after noticing that there was blood on his toothbrush after brushing. He had also seemed lethargic and had been sleeping more than usual. The physical examination revealed widespread lymphadenopathy as well as hepatosplenomegaly. The physician noted that the conjunctivas of his eyes and mucous membranes of the mouth appeared pale. Petechiae were apparent on the oral mucosa and on the undersurface of the forearm, where he was more lightly complected. The physician ordered a CBC and reticulocyte count, which gave the results shown in Table 3–9.

■ Table 3–9 ■ COMPLETE BLOOD COUNT

	Thomas H.	Childhood Reference Range[*]
WBC count	95.3	$5.5–15.5 \times 10^9$/L
RBC count	3.15	$3.9–5.3 \times 10^{12}$/L
Hb	96	115–135 g/L
Hct	.28	.34–.40 L/L
MCV	95	75–87 fL
MCH	30.5	24–30 pg
MCHC	34.0	31–37 g/dL
RDW-CV	12	12–14%[†]
Platelets	94	$150–400 \times 10^9$/L
Differential		
Neutrophils	8	41%[‡]
Bands	0	
Lymphocytes	2	50%
Monocytes	0	5%
Eosinophils	0	3%
Basophils	0	0%
Blasts	90	0%
Morphology	2 nucleated RBCs/100 WBC	
Reticulocyte count	2.8	0.5%–2.0%

[*]Handin, Lux, & Stossel, 1995.
[†]Auerbach & Alter, 1989.
[‡]Includes bands that may constitute as much as 30% of the granulocytes.

QUESTIONS

1. Describe the blood picture including WBCs, RBCs, platelets, and the differential.

2. Thomas's blood picture is characteristic of what group of conditions?

3. Based on the patient's age, what is the most likely cell line to be affected? How will the affected cell line be confirmed?

4. Discuss the classification system used for the conditions listed in question 3, including the basis for distinguishing different conditions. Also include the relative frequency of each subtype.

5. Lymphoblasts and myeloblasts are difficult to distinguish morphologically, but there are some general differences. What are they?

6. What chromosomal aberrations and mutations are seen commonly in acute lymphocytic leukemia (ALL)? Discuss any prognostic significance.

The primary care physician referred the patient to a hematology specialist, who ordered immunophenotyping. The blast cells were determined to carry the following markers:

TdT, CD22, CD10, CD19.

7. Based on the results of the immunophenotyping, what is the Revised European-American Classification of Lymphoid Neoplasms (REAL) classification of Thomas's condition?

8. What is the explanation for Thomas's anemia and thrombocytopenia?

REFERENCES

Aster, J. & Kumar, V. (1999). White cells, lymph nodes, spleen and thymus. In Cotran, R. S., Kumar, V., & Collins, T. (Eds.), *Robbins Pathologic Basis of Disease.* 6th ed. Philadelphia: W. B. Saunders.

Auerbach, A. D. & Alter, B. P. (1989). Prenatal and postnatal diagnosis of aplastic anemia. In Alter, B. P. (Ed.), *Perinatal Hematology.* London: Churchill Livingstone.

Handin, R. I., Lux, S. E. & Stossel, T. P. (Eds.) (1995). *Blood: Principles and Practice of Hematology.* Philadelphia: J. B. Lippincott.

RECOMMENDED READINGS

Bradford, C. (2000). Cytochemistry. In Rodak, B. F. (Ed.), *Hematology: Clinical Principles and Applications.* Philadelphia: W. B. Saunders.

Clare, N. & Hansen, K. (1996). Chromosome analysis of hematopoietic disorders. In McKenzie, S. B. (Ed.), *Textbook of Hematology.* 2nd ed. Baltimore: Williams & Wilkins.

Gulley, M. L. (1996). Molecular genetics of hematologic diseases. In McKenzie, S. B. (Ed.), *Textbook of Hematology.* 2nd ed. Baltimore: Williams & Wilkins.

John, K. (2000). Immunocytochemistry. In Rodak, B. F. (Ed.), *Hematology: Clinical Principles and Applications*. Philadelphia: W. B. Saunders.

Leclair, S. (2000a). Acute leukemias. In Rodak, B. F. (Ed.), *Hematology: Clinical Principles and Applications*. Philadelphia: W. B. Saunders.

Leclair, S. (2000b). Introduction to leukocyte neoplasia. In Rodak, B. F. (Ed.), *Hematology: Clinical Principles and Applications*. Philadelphia: W. B. Saunders.

McKenzie, S. B. (1996). Acute leukemias. (Ed.), In McKenzie, S. B. (Ed.), *Textbook of Hematology*. 2nd ed. Baltimore: Williams & Wilkins.

Miller, K. (2000). Molecular diagnostics. In Rodak, B. F. (Ed.), *Hematology: Clinical Principles and Applications*. Philadelphia: W. B. Saunders.

Vance, G. (2000). Cytogenetics. In Rodak, B. F. (Ed.), *Hematology: Clinical Principles and Applications*. Philadelphia: W. B. Saunders.

HEMATOLOGY CASE 3–8

John J., a 48-year-old African American man, was seen in a hospital emergency department suffering with diarrhea and vomiting, abdominal cramping, and fever that had not subsided in the past 2 days. Microbiological studies identified *Salmonella typhimurium* as the cause of the gastroenteritis. In the course of his hospitalization, a complete physical examination was conducted including routine laboratory tests. The results shown in Tables 3–10 and 3–11 prompted further investigation.

■ Table 3–10 ■ CBC AND ERYTHROCYTE SEDIMENTATION RATE

	John J.	Adult Male Reference Range*	Reference Range for Absolute Values ($\times 10^9$/L)
WBC count	11.1	5–10×10^9/L	
RBC count	2.94	5–6×10^{12}/L	
Hb	93	135–175 g/L	
Hct	.28	.41–.53 L/L	
MCV	95	80–100 fL	
MCH	31.6	26–34 pg	
MCHC	33.3	31–37 g/dL	
RDW-CV	15	11.5–14.5%	
Platelets	128	150–400×10^9/L	
Differential			
Neutrophils	32	25–60%	1.10–6.05
Bands	5	0–10%	0.10–2.1
Lymphocytes	54	20–50%	1.50–4.00
Monocytes	5	2–11%	0.20–0.95
Eosinophils	0	0–8%	0–0.70
Basophils	0	0–2%	0–0.15
Metamyelocytes	3	0	0
Plasma cells	1	0	0
Morphology	1+ toxic granulation; Döhle bodies, slight anisocytosis, rouleaux		
Westergren sedimentation rate	135	0–6 mm/h	

*Handin, Lux, & Stossel, 1995.

■ Table 3–11 ■ SELECTED CHEMISTRY PANEL RESULTS

	John J.	Reference Range
Creatinine	15	0.5–1.4 mg/dL
BUN	114	5–25 mg/dL
Total protein	12	5.5–7.5 g/dL
Albumin	2.6	3.4–4.5 g/dL
Calcium	8.2	8.5–10.5 mg/dL
Phosphorus	>10	2.5–4.5 mg/dL

QUESTIONS

1. This patient has a known bacterial infection. What findings might be expected in the CBC, and are they present?

2. a. Use proper hematologic terminology to describe the blood picture presented by John's CBC.

   b. To what conditions does a blood picture like this point?

3. What tests will be conducted to narrow the differential diagnosis, and what results are expected in each condition?

The results of these tests for this patient are shown in Tables 3–12 and 3–13.

■ Table 3–12 ■ **SPECIAL CHEMISTRY TESTS**

Serum Protein Electrophoresis	John J.	Reference Range
Total protein	11.2	5.5–7.5 g/dL
Albumin	2.8	3.4–4.5 g/dL
Alpha$_1$ globulin	0.34	0.1–0.3 g/dL
Alpha$_2$ globulin	0.78	0.5–1.0 g/dL
Beta-globulin	0.67	0.6–1.1 g/dL
Gamma	6.61	0.8–1.6 g/dL
Immunoglobulins		
IgA	< 40	88–397 mg/dL
IgM	< 35	54–220 mg/dL
IgG	6500	800–1800 mg/dL
Serum fixation electrophoresis	IgG and kappa light chains; monoclonal spike in urinary protein electrophoresis	

■ Table 3–13 ■ **BONE MARROW BIOPSY**

Uniform confluent sheet of plasma cells consisting predominantly of mononuclear cells but occasionally exhibiting binuclear plasma cells.

Myeloid and erythroid elements are virtually obliterated by the plasma cell proliferation that is also obliterating the fatty content of the marrow and thinning the oseous trabecula.

4. What diagnosis is suggested by these results?

5.   a. Describe the etiology and pathogenesis of John's condition.

b. How does this relate to the x-ray appearance of bones?

c. Which of John's test results is not typical of this condition?

6. Discuss mechanisms of immunosuppression in multiple myeloma.

7. Discuss the epidemiology of multiple myeloma.

8. What are Russell and Dutcher bodies?

9. Why is the sedimentation rate dramatically elevated in this patient?

REFERENCES

Handin, R. I., Lux, S. E. & Stossel, T. P. (Eds.). (1995). *Blood: Principles and Practice of Hematology*. Philadelphia: J. B. Lippincott.

RECOMMENDED READINGS

Aster, J. & Kumar, V. (1999). White cells, lymph nodes, spleen and thymus. In Cotran, R. S., Kumar, V., & Collins, T. (Eds.), *Robbins Pathologic Basis of Disease*. 6th ed. Philadelphia: W. B. Saunders.

Clare, N. (1996). Malignant lymphoproliferative disorders. In McKenzie, S. B. (Ed.), *Textbook of Hematology*. 2nd ed. Baltimore: Williams & Wilkins.

Clark, K. & Hippel, T. (2000). Routine testing in hematology. In Rodak, B. F. (Ed.), *Hematology: Clinical Principles and Applications*. Philadelphia: W. B. Saunders.

Johnson, M. A., Rohlfs, E. M. & Silverman, L. M. (1999). Proteins. In Burtis, C. A. & Ashwood, E. R. (Eds.), *Tietz Textbook of Clinical Chemistry*. Philadelphia: W. B. Saunders.

Kotylo, P. (2000). Lymphoproliferative disorders. In Rodak, B. F. (Ed.), *Hematology: Clinical Principles and Applications*. 3rd ed. Philadelphia: W. B. Saunders.

HEMATOLOGY CASE 3–9

Susumu H., a previously healthy 37-year-old man of Japanese descent, saw his physician, complaining of malaise, bleeding gums, and fever that had worsened over the last month. Susumu appeared pale. Splenomegaly and petechiae were detected. See Tables 3–14 and 3–15.

■ Table 3–14 ■ COMPLETE BLOOD COUNT

	Susumu H.	Adult Male Reference Range[*]
WBC count	38.1	$5–10 \times 10^9$/L
RBC count	3.20	$5–6 \times 10^{12}$/L
Hb	95	135–175 g/L
Hct	.28	.41–.53 L/L
MCV	88	80–100 fL
MCH	30	26–34 pg
MCHC	34	31–37 g/dL
RDW-CV	15	11.5–14.5%
Platelets	27	$150–400 \times 10^9$/L
Differential		
Neutrophils	3	25–60%
Bands	0	0–10%
Lymphocytes	0	20–50%
Monocytes	0	2–11%
Eosinophils	0	0–8%
Basophils	0	0–2%
Promyelocytes	39	0
Blasts	58	0
Morphology	Few Auer rods, occ. schistocyte	

[*]Handin, Lux, & Stossel, 1995.

■ Table 3–15 ■ COAGULATION TEST RESULTS

	Susumu H.	Reference Range
Prothrombin time	15	9–11 s
APTT	45	25–35 s

A bone marrow biopsy and cytochemical stains were ordered by a consulting hematologist. These showed the following:

■ Table 3–16 ■   BONE MARROW BIOPSY

Myeloblasts constituted 37% of all nucleated cells.

Promyelocytes with prominent granules constituted 23% of all nucleated cells.

Many blasts contained Auer rods, occasionally in bundles.

The blasts stained positive for myeloperoxidase and Sudan black B but negative for periodic acid-Schiff reaction.

■ Table 3–17 ■   SPECIAL TESTS

Flow cytometry for cell markers

The blast cells lack the DR(1a) antigen.

Cytogenetics

Blast cells demonstrated a t(15;17) translocation.

QUESTIONS

1. Susumu's disease is an example of what general group of hematologic disorders?

2. What classifying scheme is used for these conditions, and on what is it based?

3. Applying this classifying scheme to Susumu's test results, what condition is evident?

4. In what age groups are the acute myelogenous leukemias seen?

5. a. What chromosomal abnormality is consistently seen in this condition?

   b. What is its effect?

6. What unique treatment has been developed for this condition as a result of understanding the mutation, and what is the mechanism of its action?

7. Interpret the results of the screening hemostatis test results, and suggest further testing, especially in light of the patient's known disease.

8. Discuss the etiology of disseminated intravascular coagulation (DIC) in this condition.

9. Discuss the formation and significance of a positive test for D-dimers.

10. A bleeding time is typically part of a screening coagulation workup, yet it was not performed on this patient. Why not?

REFERENCES

Handin, R. I., Lux, S. E. & Stossel, T. P. (Eds.) (1995). *Blood: Principles and Practice of Hematology*. Philadelphia: J. B. Lippincott.

RECOMMENDED READINGS

Bradford, C. (2000). Cytochemistry. In Rodak, B. F. (Ed.), *Hematology: Clinical Principles and Applications*. Philadelphia: W. B. Saunders.

Clare, N. & Hansen, K. (1996). Chromosome analysis of hematopoietic disorders. In McKenzie, S. B. (Ed.), *Textbook of Hematology*. 2nd ed. Baltimore: Williams & Wilkins.

Gulley, M. L. (1996). Molecular genetics of hematologic diseases. In McKenzie, S. B. (Ed.), *Textbook of Hematology*. 2nd ed. Baltimore: Williams & Wilkins.

John, K. (2000). Immunocytochemistry. In Rodak, B. F. (Ed.), *Hematology: Clinical Principles and Applications*. Philadelphia: W. B. Saunders.

Leclair, S. (2000a). Acute leukemias. In Rodak, B. F. (Ed.), *Hematology: Clinical Principles and Applications*. Philadelphia: W. B. Saunders.

Leclair, S. (2000b). Introduction to leukocyte neoplasia. In Rodak, B. F. (Ed.), *Hematology: Clinical Principles and Applications*. Philadelphia: W. B. Saunders.

McKenzie, S. B. (1996). Acute leukemias. In McKenzie, S. B. (Ed.), *Textbook of Hematology*. 2nd ed. Baltimore: Williams & Wilkins.

Miller, K. (2000). Molecular diagnostics. In Rodak, B. F. (Ed.), *Hematology: Clinical Principles and Applications*. Philadelphia: W. B. Saunders.

Vance, G. (2000). Cytogenetics. In Rodak, B. F. (Ed.), *Hematology: Clinical Principles and Applications*. Philadelphia: W. B. Saunders.

HEMATOLOGY CASE 3–10

Wayne D., a 32-year-old white man, was previously healthy but recently experienced significant discomfort in his abdomen. He felt full after eating less than usual and was tired all the time. At his wife's prodding, he saw his physician because his wife thought he looked pale and that he had lost weight. The physical examination demonstrated that he had indeed lost weight and appeared pale. Splenomegaly was also detected. A CBC was ordered (see Table 3–18).

■ Table 3–18 ■   COMPLETE BLOOD COUNT

	Wayne D.	Adult Male Reference Range*	Reference Range for Absolute Values ($\times 10^9$/L)
WBC count	112	$5–10 \times 10^9$/L	
RBC count	2.10	$5–6 \times 10^{12}$/L	
Hb	70	135–175 g/L	
Hct	.20	.41–.53 L/L	
MCV	95	80–100 fL	
MCH	33	26–34 pg	
MCHC	35	31–37 g/dL	
RDW-CV	12	11.5–14.5%	
Platelets	543	$150–400 \times 10^9$/L	
Differential			
Neutrophils	35	25–60%	1.10–6.05
Bands	25	0–10%	0.10–2.1
Lymphocytes	1	20–50%	1.50–4.00
Monocytes	1	2–11%	0.20–0.95
Eosinophils	8	0–8%	0–0.70
Basophils	5	0–2%	0–0.15
Metamyelocytes	3	0	0
Myelocytes	5	0	0
Promyelocytes	10	0	0
Blasts	7	0	0
Morphology	Unremarkable		

*Handin, Lux, & Stossel, 1995.

QUESTIONS

1. Describe Wayne's blood picture using proper hematologic terminology.

2. The differential diagnosis of granulocytosis should include consideration of bacterial infection. Is this likely based on the CBC or not?

3. Considering the CBC findings and Wayne's age, what condition is most likely?

4. The promyelocytes and blasts outnumber the myelocytes and metamyelocytes. What is this called?

5. What additional testing is needed, and what results would confirm Wayne's diagnosis?

6. What is the Philadelphia chromosome, and what is its effect?

7. a. To what larger group of diseases does chronic granulocytic leukemia belong?

    b. What other diseases belong to this group, and how are they related?

REFERENCES

Handin, R. I., Lux, S. E. & Stossel, T. P. (Eds.). (1995). *Blood: Principles and Practice of Hematology*. Philadelphia: J. B. Lippincott.

RECOMMENDED READINGS

Clare, N. & Hansen, K. (1996). Molecular genetics of hematologic disease. In McKenzie, S. B. (Ed.), *Textbook of Hematology*. 2nd ed. Baltimore: Williams & Wilkins.

Leclair, S. (2000a). Chronic leukemias. In Rodak, B. F. (Ed.), *Hematology: Clinical Principles and Applications*. Philadelphia: W. B. Saunders.

Leclair, S. (2000b). Leukopoiesis. In Rodak, B. F. (Ed.), *Hematology: Clinical Principles and Applications*. Philadelphia: W. B. Saunders.

Leclair, S. (2000c). Myeloproliferative disorders. In Rodak, B. F. (Ed.), *Hematology: Clinical Principles and Applications*. Philadelphia: W. B. Saunders.

McKenzie, S. B. (1996). Myeloproliferative disorders. In McKenzie, S. B. (Ed.), *Textbook of Hematology*. 2nd ed. Baltimore: Williams & Wilkins.

Miller, K. (2000). Molecular diagnostics. In Rodak, B. F. (Ed.), *Hematology: Clinical Principles and Applications*. Philadelphia: W. B. Saunders.

4 Immunology

Bill H., a 50-year-old man, complained of morning stiffness in his joints for over a year, fatigue, and weakness. During the day, the joint pain decreased and mobility improved. His physician also noted that Bill was febrile, 100°F. The laboratory results are shown in Tables 4–1 to 4–4.

■ Table 4–1 ■ COMPLETE BLOOD COUNT

	Bill H.	Reference Range
WBC	10.2	$5–10 \times 10^9$/L
RBC	3.94	$5–6 \times 10^{12}$/L
Hemoglobin (Hb)	120	135–175 g/L
Hematocrit (Hct)	.36	.41–.53 L/L
MCV	91	80–100 fL
MCH	30	26–34 pg
MCHC	34	31–37%
Platelets	380	$150–400 \times 10^9$/L
Segmented neutrophils	85	25–60%
Band	0	0–10%
Lymphocytes	13	20–50%
Monocytes	2	2–11%
Eosinophils	0	0–8%
Basophils	0	0–2%
Atypical lymphocytes	0	0–5%
RBC morphology	Normal	Normal
ESR	40 mm/h	0–15 mm/h

Abbreviations: ESR, erythrocyte sedimentation rate; MCH, mean corpuscular hemoglobin; MCHC, mean corpuscular hemoglobin concentration; MCV, mean corpuscular volume; RBC, red blood cell; WBC, white blood cell.

■ Table 4–2 ■ CHEMISTRY TESTS

	Bill H.	Reference Range
Total protein	8.7	6.4–8.3 g/dL
Albumin	4.5	3.5–5.0 g/dL

153

■ **Table 4–3** ■   SERUM PROTEIN ELECTROPHORESIS

	Bill H.	Reference Range
Albumin	4.5	3.9–5.1 g/dL
Alpha$_1$-globulin	0.2	0.2–0.4 g/dL
Alpha$_2$-globulin	0.6	0.4–0.8 g/dL
Beta-globulin	0.9	0.5–1.0 g/dL
Gamma-globulin	2.5	0.6–1.3 g/dL

■ **Table 4–4** ■   SEROLOGY TESTS

	Bill H.	Reference Range
Rheumatoid factor (RF)	Positive	Negative
C-reactive protein	Positive	Negative
Lyme disease titer	Negative	Negative
Antinuclear antibody	40 (homogenous, diffuse)	Negative

QUESTIONS

1. Circle or highlight the abnormal results.

2. What is the probable diagnosis based on Bill's history and laboratory results?

3. What other conditions can result in a positive RF?

4. Briefly describe the RF. If the RF was negative, would you change your answer to question 2?

5. Briefly describe C-reactive protein and ESR. Are these results consistent with your diagnosis (question 2)?

6. Is a low-titer ANA consistent with your diagnosis? In other words, could patients with this condition have a positive ANA?

7. What is the epidemiology of this disease? What age groups are most likely to be affected?

8. What are the seven key symptoms established by the American College of Rheumatology?

9. Discuss two proposed etiologies (causes) of this disease.

RECOMMENDED READINGS

National Institute of Arthritis and Musculoskeletal Diseases. (1999). *Handout on Health—Rheumatoid Arthritis*. [On-line] Available: http://pharminfor.com/disease/ra/ra_handout.html [2000, August 28].

Sheehan, Catherine. (1997). *Clinical Immunology: Principles and Laboratory Diagnosis*. Philadelphia: J. B. Lippincott.

Stevens, Christine Dorresteyn. (1996). *Clinical Immunology and Serology: A Laboratory Perspective*. Philadelphia: F. A. Davis.

Turgeon, Mary Louise. (1996). *Immunology and Serology in Laboratory Medicine*. St. Louis: Mosby.

IMMUNOLOGY CASE 4-2

Mary B., a 30-year-old woman with a history of intravenous (IV) drug use, was seen at a health clinic with complaints of swollen glands, fatigue, fever, weight loss, frequent vaginal yeast infections, and a persistent skin rash that had not responded to treatment. The physician ordered the laboratory tests shown in Tables 4–5 to 4–7.

■ Table 4–5 ■   COMPLETE BLOOD COUNT

	Mary B.	Reference Range
WBC	4.0	$5–10 \times 10^9$/L
RBC	4.50	$4.0–5.0 \times 10^{12}$/L
Hb	125	120–160 g/L
Hct	.37	.36–.46 L/L
MCV	82.2	80–100 fL
MCH	28	26–34 pg
MCHC	34	31–37%
Platelets	100	$150–400 \times 10^9$/L
Segmented neutrophils	55	25–60%
Bands	0	0–10%
Lymphocytes	43	20–50%
Monocytes	2	2–11%
Eosinophils	0	0–8%
Basophils	0	0–2%
RBC morphology		Normal

■ Table 4–6 ■   CHEMISTRY

	Mary B.	Reference Range
Sodium	142	135–145 mEq/L
Potassium	3.8	3.6–5.0 mEq/L
Chloride	102	98–107 mEq/L
CO_2	30.0	24.0–34.0 mEq/L
Glucose	105	80–120 mg/dL
Bilirubin, total	0.4	0.2–1.9 mg/dL
AST	26	5–40 IU/L
ALP	53	30–157 IU/L
Total protein	6.8	6.0–8.4 g/dL
Albumin	4.0	3.5–5.2 g/dL
BUN	18	7–24 mg/dL
Creatinine	0.9	0.5–1.2 mg/dL

Abbreviations: ALP, alkaline phosphatase; AST, aspartate aminotransferase; BUN, blood urea nitrogen.

■ Table 4–7 ■ SEROLOGY

	Mary B.	Reference Range
Hepatitis serum panel		
IgM anti-HAV	Nonreactive	Nonreactive
HBsAg	Nonreactive	Nonreactive
IgM anti-HBc	Nonreactive	Nonreactive
Anti-HCV	Nonreactive	Nonreactive
HIV-ELISA	Positive	Negative

Abbreviations: ELISA, enzyme-linked immunosorbent assay; HAV, hepatitis A virus; HBcAg, hepatitis B core antigen; HbsAg, hepatitis B surface antigen; HCV, hepatitis C virus; HIV, human immunodeficiency virus, IgM, immunoglobulin M.

QUESTIONS

1. Circle or highlight the abnormal laboratory results.

2. Given Mary's physical symptoms and laboratory results, what is the probable diagnosis?

3.   a. How should the physician proceed in this case? What test(s) should be ordered?

b. What antibodies are detected in the HIV ELISA?

c. If the HIV ELISA were negative, would you change your answer to question 2?

4. What antibodies are cited in the Centers for Disease Control (CDC) criteria for the positive confirmatory test? What happens if the confirmatory test is indeterminate (does not meet all of the criteria for positivity)?

5.   a. Assuming you have been given all of the relevant medical history, in what category of this infection would this woman be classified?

b. List six conditions associated with this category.

6. List 10 conditions that are associated with the next category of this infection.

7. a. List the four primary risk factors for contracting this infection.

 b. What risk factor is the most likely cause for Mary's infection?

8. Can this infection be spread through sweat, tears, urine, or feces?

9. What test is used to monitor the progression of the disease (to categorize or stage the disease)?

10. What test is used to determine prognosis, decide on treatment and type of treatment needed, and the efficacy of treatment (response to medications)?

11. Why would the physician order a rapid plasma reagin (RPR) on this patient?

RECOMMENDED READINGS

Centers for Disease Control. (1993). *1993 Revised Classification System for HIV Infection and Expanded Surveillance Case Definition for AIDS Among Adolescents and Adults.* [On-line] Available: http://www.cdc.gov/mmwr/ preview/mmwrhtml/00018871.htm [2000, November 22].

Dubin, Jeff. (2000, July 26). *HIV Infection and AIDS.* [On-line] Available: www.emedicine.com/emerg/topic253.htm [2000, September 9].

Kuritzkes, Daniel R. (2000). *HIV Pathogenesis and Viral Markers.* [On-line] Available: www.Medscape.com/Medscape/HIV/ClinicalMgmt/CM.v02/pnt-CM.v02.html [2000, October 27].

Sheehan, Catherine. (1997). *Clinical Immunology: Principles and Laboratory Diagnosis.* Philadelphia: J. B. Lippincott.

Stevens, Christine Dorresteyn. (1996). *Clinical Immunology and Serology: A Laboratory Perspective.* Philadelphia: F. A. Davis.

Turgeon, Mary Louise. (1996). *Immunology and Serology in Laboratory Medicine.* St. Louis: Mosby.

IMMUNOLOGY CASE 4–3

Barbara F., a 30-year-old woman, presented to her physician with symptoms of weight loss, painful joints, malaise, low-grade fever, a skin rash, and swollen glands that were not painful.

Serology

Rapid plasma reagin   Positive

QUESTIONS

1. What disease/infection does the abnormal result indicate?

2. What is the causative organism? Briefly describe this organism.

3. List three other closely related species and the associated disease.

4. List and briefly discuss (include time frame and symptoms) the four stages of this disease. At what stage would she be classified?

5. What antibody is detected by the RPR? Is it specific for this disease?

6. List five conditions that are associated with biological false-positive RPRs.

7. What would the physician do next to confirm this diagnosis? Is one RPR sufficient?

8. List and briefly describe four confirmatory tests for this disease. What antibodies are detected by these tests?

9. What test is routinely used to test spinal fluid for this condition? What does this test detect?

10. Which stage of this disease can be missed by the RPR?

11. What is the treatment of choice for this condition?

RECOMMENDED READINGS

Centers for Disease Control. (1999). *Syphilis Elimination: History in the Making.* [On-line] Available: http://www.cdc.gov.nchstp/dstd/Fact_Sheets/Syphilis_Facts.htm [2000, August 11].

Sheehan, Catherine. (1997). *Clinical Immunology: Principles and Laboratory Diagnosis.* Philadelphia: J. B. Lippincott.

Stevens, Christine Dorresteyn. (1996). *Clinical Immunology and Serology: A Laboratory Perspective.* Philadelphia: F. A. Davis.

Turgeon, Mary Louise. (1996). *Immunology and Serology in Laboratory Medicine.* St. Louis: Mosby.

IMMUNOLOGY CASE 4–4

Jane C., a 38-year-old woman, visited her physician because of fatigue, fever, and joint pain (proximal interphalangeal, wrist, and knee joints). She also noticed sensitivity to the sun and reported having a rash following recent exposure. The physician noted a butterfly rash over her nose and cheeks. The laboratory results are shown in Tables 4–8 to 4–11.

■ Table 4–8 ■ COMPLETE BLOOD COUNT

	Jane C.	Reference Range[*]
WBC	4.5	$5–10 \times 10^9$/L
RBC	3.50	$4.0–5.0 \times 10^{12}$/L
Hb	105	120–160 g/L
Hct	.32	.36–.46 L/L
MCV	91.7	80–100 fL
MCH	30	26–34 pg
MCHC	33	31–37%
Platelets	100	$150–400 \times 10^9$/L
Segmented neutrophils	85	25–60%
Band	0	0–10%
Lymphocytes	13	20–50%
Monocytes	2	2–11%
Eosinophils	0	0–8%
Basophils	0	0–2%
RBC morphology		Normal

[*]Handin, Lux, & Stossel, 1995.
Abbreviations: MCHC, mean corpuscular hemoglobin concentration; MCH, mean corpuscular hemoglobin; MCV, mean corpuscular volume.

■ Table 4–9 ■ URINALYSIS

	Jane C.	Reference Range
Macroscopic		
Color	Yellow	Colorless to amber
Appearance	Cloudy, frothy	Clear
Specific gravity	1.022	1.001–1.035
pH	7.0	5–7
Protein	4+ (500 mg/dL) (SSA:4+)	Neg
Glucose	Neg	Neg
Ketones	Neg	Neg

■ **Table 4–9** ■   **URINALYSIS** *(continued)*

	Jane C.	Reference Range
Macroscopic		
Bilirubin	Neg	Neg
Blood	1+	Neg
Urobilinogen	Normal	Normal
Nitrite	Pos	Neg
Leukocyte esterase	2+	Neg
Microscopic		
WBCs	0–3/HPF	0–5/HPF
RBCs	7–10/HPF	0–2/HPF
Epithelial cells	Rare squamous/HPF	Few to moderate
	Rare renal epithelial/HPF	
Casts	0–3 hyaline/LPF	Few hyaline
	0–1 RBC/LPF	
	0–1 granular/LPF	
	0–1 waxy/LPF	

Abbreviations: SSA, sulfosalicylic acid; HPF, high-power field; LPF, low-power field.

■ **Table 4–10** ■   **CHEMISTRY TESTS**

	Jane C.	Reference Range
Sodium	140	135–145 mEq/L
Potassium	3.6	3.6–5.0 mEq/L
Chloride	106	98–107 mEq/L
CO_2	29.0	24.0–34.0 mEq/L
Glucose	116	80–120 mg/dL
Bilirubin, total	0.2	0.2–1.9 mg/dL
AST	26	5–40 IU/L
ALP	53	30–157 IU/L
Total protein	6.8	6.0–8.4 g/dL
BUN	50	7–24 mg/dL
Creatinine	2.5	0.5–1.2 mg/dL

■ **Table 4–11** ■   **SEROLOGY TESTS**

	Jane C.	Reference Range
Antinuclear Antibody	Positive 1:160	Negative
	Homogenous pattern	
Rheumatoid Factor	< 10	< 1:80 IU
C-reactive protein	3.10	< 1 mg/dL
Prealbumin	30	10–40 mg/dL

■ Table 4–11 ■   SEROLOGY TESTS (continued)

	Jane C.	Reference Range
Albumin	4000	3500–5200 mg/dL
Alpha$_1$-antitrypsin	150	115–200 mg/dL
Haptoglobin	80	40–175 mg/dL
Orosomucoid	101	55–140 mg/dL
Alpha$_2$-macroglobulin	205	130–300 mg/dL
Transferrin	300	215–380 mg/dL
Complement C3	50	83–177 mg/dL
Complement C4	20	29–68 mg/dL
Immunoglobulin G	3020	565–1765 mg/dL
Immunoglobulin A	330	40–350 mg/dL
Immunoglobulin M	420	50–300 mg/dL
Apolipoprotein B	99	63–133 mg/dL
Apolipoprotein A	103	94–178 mg/dL
Iron	80	65–175 µg/dL
% Transferrin saturation	25	20–50%

QUESTIONS

1. Circle or highlight the abnormal laboratory results.

2. Given Jane's physical symptoms, list four conditions that should be ruled out (or in).

3. After reviewing the results of the physical examination and laboratory results, what is the most probable diagnosis?

4. Briefly describe the pathophysiology of this disease. What is happening in Jane's body?

5. If the rheumatoid factor were positive, would you change your answer to question 3? Why or why not?

6.   a. List the 11 criteria proposed by the American College of Rheumatology for diagnosing this condition.

      b. How many are needed for a diagnosis?

7. How many of the criteria listed in question 6 has Jane experienced?

8. Describe or define antinuclear antibody (ANA). List five different types of ANAs.

9. What two ANAs are specific for this condition?

10. What is the significance of the abnormal urinalysis and chemistry tests?

11. Are the complement levels consistent with your diagnosis? If yes, why?

12. List and briefly describe four factors that *may* play a role in systemic lupus erythematosus (SLE).

RECOMMENDED READINGS

Sheehan, Catherine. (1997). *Clinical Immunology: Principles and Laboratory Diagnosis*. Philadelphia: J. B. Lippincott.

Stevens, Christine Dorresteyn. (1996). *Clinical Immunology and Serology: A Laboratory Perspective*. Philadelphia: F. A. Davis.

Turgeon, Mary Louise. (1996). *Immunology and Serology in Laboratory Medicine*. St. Louis: Mosby.

WebMD. (1999). *Systemic Lupus Erythematosus*. [On-line] Available: http://webmed.lycos.com/content/dmk/dmk_article_40056 [2000, October 3].

IMMUNOLOGY CASE 4–5

Tammy R., an 18-year-old college freshman, went to the University Health Center complaining of a sore throat, fever, and exhaustion. The physician noted swollen lymph glands and ordered a complete blood count (CBC); chemistry profile, strep screen, and monotest. See Tables 4–12 and 4–13.

■ **Table 4–12** ■   **CBC**

	Tammy R.	Reference Range[*]
WBC	14.5	$5–10 \times 10^9$/L
RBC	5.35	$4.0–5.0 \times 10^{12}$/L
Hb	148	120–160 g/L
Hct	.45	.36–.46 L/L
MCV	84	80–100 fL
MCH	28	26–34 pg
MCHC	33	31–37%
Platelets	225	150–400 mm³
Segmented neutrophils	28	25–60%
Band	0	0–10%
Lymphocytes	40	20–50%
Monocytes	6	2–11%
Eosinophils	0	0–8%
Basophils	1	0–2%
Atypical lymphocytes	25	0–5%
RBC morphology		Normal

[*]Handin, Lux, & Stossel, 1995.

■ **Table 4–13** ■   **CHEMISTRY RESULTS**

	Tammy R.	Reference Range
Chemistry		
Sodium	141	136–145 mEq/L
Potassium	4.4	3.6–5.0 mEq/L
Chloride	107	101–111 mEq/L
CO_2	27.0	24.0–34.0 mEq/L
Glucose	92	80–120 mg/dL
Bilirubin total	1.9	0.2–1.2 mg/dL
AST	89	5–40 IU/L
ALT	80	6–37 IU/L
Total protein	6.5	6.0–8.4 g/dL
BUN	15	7–24 mg/dL
Creatinine	0.9	0.5–1.2 mg/dL

■ Table 4–13 ■   CHEMISTRY RESULTS *(continued)*

	Tammy R.	Reference Range
Calcium	8.8	8.5–10.5 mg/dL
Albumin	3.9	3.5–5.0 g/dL
Serology and Microbiology Results		
Serology	Monotest	Positive
Microbiology	Strep screen	Negative

Abbreviation: ALT, alanine aminotransferase.

QUESTIONS

1. What are the abnormal laboratory results?

2. Based on Tammy's history (symptoms) and laboratory results, what is the probable diagnosis?

3. What age group is associated with this disease? Why is it known as the "kissing disease"?

4. If the monotest were negative, would you change your answer to question 2? Explain why or why not.

5. What antibodies react in the monotest?

6. a. List and briefly describe three classes of antibodies making up this group of antibodies.

   b. Briefly explain the Davidsohn differential test.

   c. Briefly describe the monotest.

7. What virus is usually associated with this disease? What other diseases are also associated with this virus?

8.   a. What would the physician do next?

     b. If it is still negative, what test(s) can be ordered to confirm the diag-
        nosis?

9.   a. What viral antibodies or antigens are commonly available?

     b. At what stage of this disease are they found?

10. What other viruses are also associated with this disease?

11. What other more serious, life-threatening diseases must be ruled out?

12.   a. What organ system is associated with the abnormal chemistry tests?

      b. Is this consistent with your original diagnosis?

13. What is the usual course of this disease: incubation period and time to recover?

14. What is the normal treatment for this disease?

RECOMMENDED READINGS

Centers for Disease Control. (1999). *Epstein-Barr Virus and Infectious Mononucleosis*. [On-line] Available: http://www.cdc.gov/nciod/diseases/ebv.htm [2000, August 9].

Sheehan, Catherine. (1997). *Clinical Immunology: Principles and Laboratory Diagnosis*. Philadelphia: J. B. Lippincott.

Stevens, Christine Dorresteyn. (1996). *Clinical Immunology and Serology: A Laboratory Perspective*. Philadelphia: F. A. Davis.

Turgeon, Mary Louise. (1996). *Immunology and Serology in Laboratory Medicine*. St. Louis: Mosby.

5 Microbiology

Frank J. Scarano, Ph.D.

A 75-year-old man, Patrick R., presented to the emergency room with fever, shortness of breath, chest pain, and severe, extremely productive cough. Patrick had been a heavy smoker for almost 50 years before he quit 7 years ago, when he was diagnosed with emphysema. Patrick occasionally used oxygen at home when he had difficulty breathing, and on presentation he was using portable oxygen because of his severe respiratory distress. A chest x-ray revealed a right lower lobe infiltrate, and Patrick was admitted to the hospital. Sputum, urine, and blood cultures were collected.

The direct Gram's stain of the sputum specimen revealed the following:

Many neutrophils (>25 per low-power field)

Rare squamous epithelial cells (<1 per-low-power field)

Many gram-positive lancet-shaped diplococci and cocci in short chains (>25 per oil immersion field)

Few gram-negative diplococci (<10 per oil immersion field)

Few gram-positive bacilli (<10 per oil immersion field)

After overnight incubation at 35°C in 5% to 7% CO_2, a blood-agar plate inoculated with the specimen revealed a mixture of two colony types. Rare, non-hemolytic, tiny, white, dry-looking colonies were present. A predominance of small, wet-looking, convex (crater-form), entire-edged colonies were also seen, with a greening of the medium around them.

The urine culture showed no growth at 24 hours. All blood cultures were negative after 5 days' incubation.

QUESTIONS

1. Based on the direct Gram's stain, what is the quality of this sputum specimen? Is this specimen of acceptable quality to provide clinically relevant information?

2. Based on the colony morphology and the Gram's stain, what organism is suspect as the cause of Patrick's pneumonia?

3. What type of hemolysis is being described by the term "greening" of the medium?

4. What other (nonpathogenic) organisms commonly found in this type of specimen also cause this type of hemolysis?

5. What laboratory tests are useful in differentiating these organisms and identifying the pathogen? List at least two tests, and be sure to include expected reactions for each organism.

6. Organisms other than the predominant organism were seen in the Gram's stain and culture. Does this mean that the patient has a polymicrobial pneumonia? Why are those other organisms present?

7. Should antimicrobial susceptibility testing be performed on this pathogen? If so, what antimicrobial agent(s) should be tested? If not, why not?

8. What virulence factor does the pathogen possess that can help it evade the host's defense mechanisms?

9. What preventative measures can be used to prevent infection or reinfection with this pathogen?

10. In this case, the symptoms were quite diagnostic of pneumonia. Why were urine and blood cultures also collected?

RECOMMENDED READINGS

Koneman, Elmer W., et al. (1997). *Color Atlas and Textbook of Diagnostic Microbiology*. 5th ed. Philadelphia: J. B. Lippincott.

Mahon, Connie R. & Manuselis, George. (1995). *Textbook of Diagnostic Microbiology*. Philadelphia: W. B. Saunders.

Murray, Patrick R., et al. (1995). *Manual of Clinical Microbiology*. 6th ed. Washington D.C.: ASM Press.

MICROBIOLOGY CASE 5–2

A 47-year-old married man, Mike A., reported to a local clinic with complaints of slight chest pain, shortness of breath, dysuria (difficult, painful urination), and a milky-white urethral discharge. His previous medical history was significant for hypercholesterolemia and hypertension. These conditions were being managed with diet and exercise and continued to be monitored by his regular physician. Mike was proud to announce that he had lost 30 pounds over the past year and had been working out regularly at the gym. He mentioned that he had been feeling very well, "like I was 25 years old again," until 3 days ago, when the dysuria and discharge first started. He admitted that he did not want to visit his regular physician because of the nature of this problem but was starting to become increasingly anxious about his situation. Mike divulged further that he had been having an affair with a woman he met at the gym. They had been sexually intimate over the past 6 weeks, and they had unprotected intercourse a week ago. A urethral specimen was collected for routine sexually transmitted disease (STD) workup, and Mike was treated empirically with antibiotics.

Direct Gram's stain of the urethral discharge revealed many polymorphonuclear leukocytes and numerous intra- and extra-cellular coffee bean-shaped gram-negative diplococci.

QUESTIONS

1. Based on the Gram's stain results, what organism do you suspect is causing Mike's infection?

2. What considerations should be made for appropriate specimen transport for these types of specimens?

3. "Routine" STD workups may consist of molecular diagnostic techniques, conventional culture methods, or both. If the specimen is processed for conventional culture, what type(s) of media would be appropriate for recovery of the organism responsible for this man's infection? Be sure to mention the important components of the media and their purpose, as well as any specialized inoculation techniques and the appropriate atmosphere of incubation.

4. What subsequent testing would be appropriate for identification of the organism?

5. What are some of the key biochemical characteristics that are useful in identifying this organism?

6. Describe the molecular diagnostic techniques that may also be used to identify this organism and another etiologic agent in STD.

7. What would be an advantage to using molecular diagnostic techniques in this situation?

8. What might be a disadvantage to using these techniques?

9. What does *empiric* mean?

10. What antimicrobial chemotherapy would be appropriate for Mike?

11. What should be done about the woman from the gym and Mike's wife?

RECOMMENDED READINGS

Koneman, Elmer W., et al. (1997). *Color Atlas and Textbook of Diagnostic Microbiology*. 5th ed. Philadelphia: J. B. Lippincott.

Murray, Patrick R., et al. (1995). *Manual of Clinical Microbiology*. 6th ed. Washington D.C.: ASM Press.

MICROBIOLOGY CASE 5-3

A 16-year-old cystic fibrosis patient, Ellen J., reported to her pulmonologist for a routine visit. Ellen mentioned that for the most part she had been feeling well except that she had been feeling somewhat lethargic for the past 2 days. She said that she felt slightly feverish yesterday, but she did not feel feverish today. Her current temperature was recorded as 99.1°F. Her pulse and blood pressure were within normal limits, and her weight was holding steady relative to her previous visit. Her respirations were slightly rapid and shallow, although she did not feel short of breath. As is the standard practice for her visits, expectorated respiratory secretions were collected and sent to the laboratory for culture.

Direct Gram's stain revealed:

Few neutrophils (1 to 9 per low-power field)
Moderate squamous epithelial cells (10 to 24 per low-power field)
Moderate (10 to 24 per oil immersion field) gram-positive cocci in chains
Moderate gram-positive cocci in clusters
Moderate gram-negative cocci
Moderate gram-positive (diphtheroid) bacilli
Few (1 to 9 per oil immersion field) gram-negative bacilli

After appropriate incubation, abundant growth was observed on the nonselective media. The colony characteristics on trypticase soy agar plus 5% sheep blood (blood agar plate) included the following: pinpoint-to-small alpha-hemolytic colonies, small gray gamma-hemolytic colonies, medium-sized smooth cream-to-white–colored colonies, small clear/translucent wet-looking colonies, small rough "crunchy" white colonies, and occasional large gray mucoid colonies. The selective media showed only one colony morphology: large, mucoid, lactose-negative colonies. Specialized selective and differential media showed large, very mucoid, yellow colonies.

QUESTIONS

1. Based on the direct Gram's stain, what is the quality of this sputum specimen? Is this specimen acceptable for further processing (plating/ planting)?

2. What types of media would be appropriate for processing routine sputum specimens, and what additional media are recommended for processing sputum specimens from cystic fibrosis patients?

3. Why are these routine and special media used for sputum specimens?

4. What atmosphere of incubation is suggested for these plates?

5. How should the screening of the nonselective media proceed? Be sure to indicate suspect upper respiratory flora, suspected pathogens, and appropriate screening tests or identification methods in your answer.

6. How should the workup of the selective media proceed?

RECOMMENDED READINGS

Koneman, Elmer W., et al. (1997). *Color Atlas and Textbook of Diagnostic Microbiology.* 5th ed. Philadelphia: J. B. Lippincott.

Mahon, Connie R. & Manuselis, George. (1995). *Textbook of Diagnostic Microbiology.* Philadelphia: W. B. Saunders.

Murray, Patrick R., et al. (1995). *Manual of Clinical Microbiology.* 6th ed. Washington D.C.: ASM Press.

MICROBIOLOGY CASE 5–4

Jack and Diane R., a 25-year-old newlywed couple, reported to the emergency room with abdominal pain and diarrhea of 4 days' duration. They stated that they initially thought they "picked up a summer stomach flu" because they recently returned from a 5-day camping trip. Jack added, "We were really roughin' it Doc. It was great until the weather got miserable, rainy, and cold the last 2 days of the trip!"

The symptoms began shortly after their return and included fever, headache, myalgia, and malaise. The diarrhea started the next day and was mild at first with 2 to 3 loose bowel movements per day. The diarrhea became more severe and was up to 7 to 9 watery bowel movements per day with severe cramping. The physician asked many questions about the trip to collect a complete history. The couple denied drinking any water from the lake near their campsite, although after further questioning they admitted to skinny-dipping in the lake one evening "before the weather got bad." Diane mentioned that although this trip was Jack's idea of "roughin' it" they were careful to use only bottled water for drinking. She went on to explain that they bathed and used the sanitary facilities provided at the campsite and used only potable water from that facility for washing dishes and cooking. They described the food they had eaten during their trip, including hamburgers, hot dogs, chicken, roasted corn, canned beans, macaroni salad, and cole slaw (cabbage salad). They transported the meat frozen and were careful to keep all the food on ice as much as possible. Diane mentioned that she thought the chicken they ate for lunch their last day may have been undercooked, but she did not want to make Jack go back out into the rain to cook it longer.

Physical examinations of both Jack and Diane were unremarkable except for slight dehydration and elevated temperature (Jack 100.9°F, Diane 100.2°F). Both patients had slight diffuse abdominal tenderness upon palpation. Stool specimens were collected from both patients and processed for ova and parasite examination. Routine stool culture for bacterial pathogens was also ordered.

Parasitology report: "No ova or parasites seen."

Observation of the bacteriology plates showed many lactose-positive organisms on the gram-negative selective agar. Specialized selective media had only rare colonies of lactose-positive organisms in the area of the primary inoculum. The CAMPY agar plate showed moderate growth.

QUESTIONS

1. Why might the physician suspect that parasites could be a possibility in these patients?

2. What parasites might the physician have suspected?

3. How should a stool culture for routine bacterial pathogens be processed? Be sure to include appropriate media and atmosphere of incubation.

4. What bacterial pathogens should be included in the screening of a routine stool culture, and how would the clinical laboratory scientist processing the culture recognize these potential pathogens?

5. When a stool specimen is bloody, additional testing is often recommended or suggested to the physician (especially with children or the elderly). What pathogen is of concern in that situation, and how is this specimen processed?

6. Other more unusual bacterial pathogens may also cause diarrheal disease, and physicians may request additional testing for these organisms. What organisms might be suspected, and what media and atmosphere of incubation are used to isolate these organisms?

7. Based on the history and laboratory results presented, what is the most probable cause for the diarrheal disease in these patients?

RECOMMENDED READINGS

Koneman, Elmer W., et al. (1997). *Color Atlas and Textbook of Diagnostic Microbiology*. 5th ed. Philadelphia: J. B. Lippincott.

Mahon, Connie R. & Manuselis, George. (1995). *Textbook of Diagnostic Microbiology*. Philadelphia: W. B. Saunders.

Mandell, Gerald L., et al. (2000). *Mandell, Douglas, and Bennett's Principles and Practice of Infectious Diseases*. 5th ed., vols. 1 & 2. Philadelphia: Churchill Livingstone.

Murray, Patrick R., et al. (1995). *Manual of Clinical Microbiology*, 6th ed. Washington D.C.: ASM Press.

MICROBIOLOGY CASE 5–5

A 33-year-old pregnant woman, Stephanie D., reported to the emergency department with premature labor. She stated that she had been feeling a little "under the weather" for the past week with slight fever, some back pain, and headache. She explained that she began to feel "some occasional crampiness" over the previous 24 hours but did not think this could be contractions because she was only 30 weeks' pregnant. She was surprised with membrane rupture about 2 hours ago and had experienced an increase in frequency of the contractions, which were now approximately 3 minutes apart. She was taken to the delivery room and eventually delivered a 950-gram boy. The infant was in severe respiratory distress and was intubated immediately. Gross examination of the placenta revealed ischemic areas, and samples of the tissue were sent to pathology and microbiology. Cerebrospinal fluid (CSF) and blood cultures from the baby were also collected.

Results

Direct Gram's stain of the CSF revealed many neutrophils and short gram-positive coccobacilli. The pathology examination showed multiple abscesses approximately 1 to 3 cm in diameter. Upon microscopic examination, the abscesses revealed neutrophilic infiltration and aggregates of necrotic villi. Placental tissue, CSF, and blood cultures were all positive within 24 hours. The colonies on blood-agar plate (BAP) were small, translucent, and gray with a very narrow zone of beta-hemolysis. (The microbiologist did not even notice the hemolysis until she had removed a colony for further testing.) Further testing included a positive catalase test, an umbrella-like zone of growth in motility media at 22°C, growth at 4°C, a positive esculin hydrolysis test, and a negative H_2S reaction.

QUESTIONS

1. What organism is likely to have caused Stephanie's premature labor and infection of the neonate?

2. The causative agent of this infection can be confused with *Streptococcus agalactiae*, which can also be pathogenic in this setting. How are these two organisms similar, and what laboratory tests are helpful in distinguishing the two?

3. No history was presented that elucidated the source of Stephanie's infection. How might one become infected with the causative organism?

4. Why is the ability of this organism to grow at 4°C important to its pathogenicity?

5. What measures should be taken to avoid infection with this organism?

6. Pregnant women are predisposed to infection with this organism. What other groups are at high risk?

7. What are some of the virulence factors this organism possesses?

RECOMMENDED READINGS

Broome, C. V. (1993). Listeriosis: Can we prevent it? *ASM News* 59:444–446.

Koneman, Elmer W., et al. (1997). *Color Atlas and Textbook of Diagnostic Microbiology*. 5th ed. Philadelphia: J. B. Lippincott.

Mandell, Gerald L., et al. (2000). *Mandell, Douglas, and Bennett's Principles and Practice of Infectious Diseases*. 5th ed., vol. 2. Philadelphia: Churchill Livingstone.

Murray, Patrick R., et al. (1999). *Manual of Clinical Microbiology*. 7th ed. Washington D.C.: ASM Press.

MICROBIOLOGY CASE 5–6

A 59-year-old man, Fred C., presented to the emergency room complaining of fever and chills of 4 days' duration, with dizziness over the last 24 hours. He also complained of intermittent diarrhea and constipation over the past 6 months with occasional bloody stool. Fred had been a heavy smoker of 45 years and admitted to drinking alcohol regularly, "Two or three beers a night." The patient's breathing was rapid, but his lung sounds were clear. His temperature was recorded as 102.3°C. Fred was hypotensive, tachycardic, and had an appreciable heart murmur. Blood was drawn for a complete blood count (CBC) and culture. A stool specimen was collected to test for occult blood, and a chest x-ray was performed.

Results of the laboratory tests are shown in Table 5–1 and in the following list.

■ Table 5–I ■   HEMATOLOGY RESULTS

| | Complete Blood Count | |
	Fred C.	Reference Range
WBC	9.1	$5–10 \times 10^9$/L
RBC	4.00	$5–6 \times 10^{12}$/L
Hb	122	135–180 g/L
Hct	.40	.41–.53 L/L
MCV	100	80–100 fL
MCH	32	26–34 pg
MCHC	30	31–37%
RDW	15.6	11.0–14.5
Platelets	458	$150–400 \times 10^9$/L
MPV	7.2 fL	6.5–12.0 fL
RBC morphology	2+ microcytosis	
	1+ macrocytosis	
	1+ ovalocytosis	
	1+ basophilic stipling	
	2+ hypochromia	
	1+ polychromatophilia	
	2+ toxic granulation	
	Rare Döhle bodies	
	Rare hypersegmentation	
	2 nucleated RBCs	

| | Differential | |
	Fred C.	Reference Range
Polymorphonuclear neutrophils	52	25–60%
Bands	10	0–10%
Lymphocytes	35	20–50%

[handwritten marginalia: "slight anemia ↗ correlate", "↗ NRBC ↗ correlate", "toxic gran", "Döhle bodies", "correlate", "metamyelocyte"]

■ **Table 5–1** ■   **HEMATOLOGY RESULTS** *(continued)*

| | *Differential* | |
	Fred C.	*Reference Range*
Monocytes	1	2–11%
Metamyelocytes	2	0%

Abbreviations: Hb, hemoglobin; Hct, Hematocrit; MCH, mean corpuscular hemoglobin; MCHC, mean corpuscular hemoglobin concentration; MCV, mean corpuscular volume; MPV, mean platelet volume; RBC, red blood cell; RDW, red blood cell distribution width index; WBC, white blood cell.

The stool was positive for occult blood.

All blood cultures were positive within 24 hours

Gram's stains from the bottles revealed gram-positive cocci in chains.

Subcultures grew readily on BAP and produced small gray gamma-hemolytic colonies.

Additional biochemical testing yielded the following: catalase, negative; bile esculine agar, growth with black precipitate; growth in 6.5% NaCl, negative; L-Pyrrolidonyl β-naphthylamide PYR test, negative.

QUESTIONS

1. What would be the appropriate timing and number for the collection of routine blood cultures?

2. Because of the sensitivity of blood cultures, contamination can be a problem. What step(s) should be followed to keep the contamination rate low?

3. What criteria might be used to determine if a positive blood culture is due to contamination or bacteremia?

4. Does Fred have bacteremia? Does Fred have septicemia? What is the difference between bacteremia and septicemia?

5. Given the Gram's stain reaction and morphology of the bacteria recovered from these blood cultures, what might be some possibilities for the identity of the organism?

6. Given Fred's history, physical findings, other clinical data, and the further biochemical testing that was performed on this isolate, what is the likely identification of this organism?

7. If latex agglutination testing was performed, to which group would this organism belong?

8. What other testing methods might be employed to get a definitive identification of this organism by genus and species?

9. Complete identification of this organism from blood culture may be very helpful to the physician because of the association of this organism with specific medical conditions. Although Fred has multiple underlying medical problems, with which condition is this organism often associated?

REFERENCES

Leclair, Susan J. (2000). Personal communication, University of Massachusetts, Dartmouth.

RECOMMENDED READINGS

Koneman, Elmer W., et al. (1997). *Color Atlas and Textbook of Diagnostic Microbiology*. 5th ed. Philadelphia: J. B. Lippincott.

Mandell, Gerald L., et al. (2000). *Mandell, Douglas, and Bennett's Principles and Practice of Infectious Diseases*. 5th ed. Philadelphia: Churchill Livingstone.

Murray, Patrick R., et al. (1995). *Manual of Clinical Microbiology*. 6th ed. Washington D.C.: ASM Press.

MICROBIOLOGY CASE 5-7

An 18-month-old boy, Bobby H., was rushed to the emergency room by ambulance after his mother found him unresponsive. When he did not wake up at his usual time from a nap, she became concerned. When she tried to wake him, he would not respond and is currently lethargic and listless. His mother reported that he had had a fever for 2 days and had been cranky and irritable. The mother stated, "I think he might have an earache, because he started pulling at his ear yesterday." The family is from an extremely rural area and does not have medical insurance or easy access to health clinics. Bobby had not had any routine pediatric well-care visits or immunizations. Bobby's temperature was 39.5°C. A lumbar puncture was performed and revealed the following: CSF protein, 989 mg/dL (normal, 15 to 45 mg/dL); glucose, 12 mg/dL (normal, 40 to 80 mg/dL); 20,000 WBC/mm^3 with 90% polymorphonuclear cells. Gram's stain of the CSF showed gram-negative pleomorphic coccobacilli and many neutrophils. The spinal fluid culture yielded abundant growth on chocolate agar after overnight incubation. The colonies are small, round, and translucent with a glistening/wet appearance. The microbiologist working up the culture recognized a familiar mousy odor to the culture.

QUESTIONS

1. What organism is most likely causing Bobby's infection?

2. What special growth requirements does this organism exhibit, and how can these be used to help identify the organism?

3. What methods might be used to test for these growth requirements?

4. Even without the Gram's stain or culture, how do the CSF parameters point toward a bacterial disease?

5. What other bacteria commonly cause this disease in this age group?

6. Latex agglutination testing is available for this and some of the other pathogens. When would this type of testing be appropriate?

7. How can infection with this organism be prevented?

RECOMMENDED READINGS

Koneman, Elmer W., et al. (1997). *Color Atlas and Textbook of Diagnostic Microbiology*. 5th ed. Philadelphia: J. B. Lippincott.

Mandell, Gerald L., et al. (2000). *Mandell, Douglas, and Bennett's Principles and Practice of Infectious Diseases*. 5th ed., vols. 1 & 2. Philadelphia: Churchill Livingstone.

Murray, Patrick R., et al. (1999). *Manual of Clinical Microbiology*. 7th ed. Washington D.C.: ASM Press.

MICROBIOLOGY CASE 5–8

An observant microbiologist noticed that in the past 2 days, three patients from the orthopedic unit of the hospital had all had wound infections with the same organism and that organism had an unusual antibiogram (antimicrobial sensitivity pattern).

Patient 1, Paula C., an 88-year-old woman, had total hip replacement surgery 5 days ago. Her past medical history was significant for hypertension and geriatric hyperthyroidism. Her thyroid was inactivated 12 years ago, and she had been on synthetic hormone replacement medication since then. Her hypertension was also regulated with medication, and her blood pressure was monitored regularly. Two days ago, a purulent discharge was noticed at the surgical site, and a specimen was collected for culture and sensitivity. The direct Gram's stain of a specimen from the surgical wound yielded many neutrophils, rare squamous epithelial cells, RBCs, and numerous gram-positive cocci in clusters.

Patient 2, William M., a 27-year-old man, had femur reconstruction 6 days ago, secondary to a motor vehicle accident. His past medical history was unremarkable. Three days ago, his surgical site appeared red and inflamed, and a significant quantity of purulent, sanguineous discharge was present. The exudate was collected for culture and sensitivity. The direct Gram's stain of a specimen from the surgical wound yielded moderate neutrophils, no squamous epithelial cells, and numerous gram-positive cocci in clusters.

Patient 3, Ronald T., a 34-year-old man, had outpatient arthroscopic surgery on his left knee 5 days ago. Ronald was an avid amateur athlete whose medical history was significant only for chronic knee injuries over the past 12 years. Ronald's initial surgery appeared to have gone well, and he was discharged after several hours, as is usual for this type of surgery. However, he reported to the emergency room 2 days ago with fever and pain and swelling of the knee. Blood cultures were collected, and a sample of the exudate from his knee was also submitted to the laboratory for Gram's stain and culture. Due to the systemic nature of Ronald's infection, he was admitted and empiric intravenous antibiotic therapy was initiated. The direct Gram's stain of the exudate yielded numerous neutrophils, rare squamous epithelial cells, and many gram-positive cocci in clusters. All three sets of blood cultures were positive within 24 hours with gram-positive cocci in clusters.

The isolates from all three patients were round, medium-sized, cream-colored, beta-hemolytic colonies on BAP. The isolates were catalase positive and coagulase positive. The isolates grew readily on oxacillin screening media, and antimicrobial susceptibility testing revealed resistance to oxacillin.

QUESTIONS

1. Based on the data presented, what organism is causing these surgical wound infections?

2. What other tests, in addition to those listed here, could be useful in the identification of this organism?

3. What special conditions should be employed when performing antimicrobial susceptibility testing on this organism?

4. What would be the appropriate therapy for these patients?

5. What general term is used to describe infections that are acquired while the patient is in a hospital or other institutional setting?

6. What is the single most effective means of preventing the spread of infection?

7. It is possible that these infections were caused by the same organism, perhaps spread in the unit by an individual or an inanimate object. What techniques could be employed to determine if these isolates are of the same strain?

RECOMMENDED READINGS

Koneman, Elmer W., et al. (1997). *Color Atlas and Textbook of Diagnostic Microbiology*. 5th ed. Philadelphia: J. B. Lippincott.

Mandell, Gerald L., et al. (2000). *Mandell, Douglas, and Bennett's Principles and Practice of Infectious Diseases*. 5th ed., vols. 1 & 2. Philadelphia: Churchill Livingstone.

Murray, Patrick R., et al. (1999). *Manual of Clinical Microbiology*. 7th ed. Washington D.C.: ASM Press.

MICROBIOLOGY CASE 5–9

A 21-year-old female student, Maria P., reported to the University Health Office with a complaint of diarrhea and severe flatulence of 9 days' duration. She also reported anorexia, malaise, abdominal bloating, and cramping with nausea. A complete physical and history were performed. The physical examination revealed an otherwise healthy young woman with a slight heart murmur. The murmur was first discovered when she was a young child and is considered a minor congenital defect. The murmur did not interfere with her living an active life, and no therapy was required. Her physical also revealed that she had lost 13 pounds since her last visit. Maria indicated that this was not due to dieting, but rather to the fact that she had been feeling very ill lately and that she "hadn't eaten much" in the past week and a half. The history revealed that the student was a biology major who returned 3 weeks ago from an externship at a beaver sanctuary in rural Colorado. She was a research assistant involved in a study that required fieldwork at the beaver dams, with regular handling of the animals to monitor weight and other parameters. She had also traveled to Portugal with her parents 9 months ago to visit her grandparents and extended family. She had a 6-year-old Great Dane and two cats but no "exotic" pets. Maria had no allergies, and she did not regularly take any medications, although she did take a daily multivitamin with iron. She also admitted that when she first started feeling ill she "took some antibiotic that was left over from when I had Strep throat 2 years ago."

Stools were collected for routine culture, ova and parasite analysis, and *Clostridium difficile* toxin assay. Laboratory results were as follows:

C. difficile toxin assay was negative.

Stool culture: "No *Salmonella* spp., *Shigella* spp., or *Campylobacter* spp. isolated, please consult laboratory if other enteric bacterial pathogens are suspected."

The ova and parasite examination was positive for characteristic cysts in the concentrate and for trophozoites in the permanent stained smear. The cysts were thin-walled, smooth, oval-shaped, and approximately 8 to 12 µm long and 7 to 10 µm wide. The cysts were quite refractile, and some demonstrated centrally located bands and two eccentrically located nuclei. The trophozoites were approximately 10 to 20 µm long and 5 to 10 µm wide. The trophozoites also showed centrally located dark bands and two eccentrically located nuclei, each with a prominent central karyosome. The arrangement of the nuclei and dark bands created an "old-man face"-like image.

QUESTIONS

1. Based on Maria's history, presentation, and the description of the organism, what parasite is causing the problem?

2. What was significant from Maria's history that would make the physician suspect this pathogen?

3. What term is used for the centrally located bands often seen in this organism?

4. What other intestinal parasite(s) might the physician have suspected?

5. What are the recommended timing and number of specimens for diagnosis of intestinal parasites?

6. Traditional methods for ova and parasite examination include a concentrate and permanent stained slide. Why are both methods suggested?

7. What disease process did the physician suspect when the *C. difficile* toxin assay was ordered?

8. What was significant from Maria's history that would make the physician suspect this disease?

9. Describe the *C. difficile* toxin assay.

10. Why is *C. difficile* toxin assay favored over culture as a method to diagnose this disease?

RECOMMENDED READINGS

Mahon, Connie R. & Manuselis, George. (1995). *Textbook of Diagnostic Microbiology*. Philadelphia: W. B. Saunders.

Mandell, Gerald L., et al., (2000). *Mandell, Douglas, and Bennett's Principles and Practice of Infectious Diseases*. 5th ed., vols. 1 & 2. Philadelphia: Churchill Livingstone.

Murray, Patrick R., et al. (1999). *Manual of Clinical Microbiology*. 7th ed. Washington D.C.: ASM Press.

MICROBIOLOGY CASE 5–10

A 73-year-old man, Elmer W., reported to his physician with complaints of fever, nausea, and abdominal pain and tenderness of 2 days' duration. Elmer was a chronic diabetic with end-stage renal disease. His diabetes was being regulated with insulin injections and diet. His kidney disease was being treated with continuous ambulatory peritoneal dialysis (CAPD). On examination, Elmer was tachycardic and had a temperature of 103.6°F. Before dialysis, blood was drawn for CBC, routine chemistry analysis, and culture. A sample of CAPD fluid was also collected for routine culture and sensitivity testing. See Tables 5–2 to 5–4.

■ Table 5–2 ■ HEMATOLOGY RESULTS

	CBC	
	Elmer W.	*Reference Range*
WBC	9.5	$5–10 \times 10^9/L$
RBC	3.29	$5–6 \times 10^{12}/L$
Hb	98	135–180 g/L
Hct	.31	.41–.53 L/L
MCV	95	80–100 fL
MCH	30	26–34 pg
MCHC	31	31–37%
RDW	14.8	11.0–14.5
Platelets	202	$150–400 \times 10^9/L$
MPV	6.5–12.0 fL	
RBC morphology:	1+ microcytes	
	1+ macrocytes	
	2+ target cells	
	1+ burr cells	

	Differential	
	Elmer W.	*Reference Range*
Polymorphonuclear neutrophils	77	25–60%
Bands	3	0–10%
Lymphocytes	18	20–50%
Monocytes	2	2–11%

■ Table 5–3 ■ CHEMISTRY RESULTS

	Elmer W.	*Reference Range*
ALT	88	6–37 U/L
ALP	101	30–90 U/L
Cholesterol	245	< 200 mg/dL
Triglycerides	320	67–157 mg/dL

■ Table 5–3 ■ CHEMISTRY RESULTS (continued)

	Elmer W.	Reference Range
Chloride	107	95–105 mEq/L
Amylase	301	95–290 U/L
Lipase	2.2	0.5–1.2 U/L
Random glucose	246	65–110 mg/dL
Total protein	5.0	6.0–8.0 g/dL
Albumin	1.9	2.6–5.2 g/dL
BUN	85	5–20 mg/dL
Creatinine	5.8	< 1.2 mg/dL
Potassium	6.0	3.5–5.0 mEq/L
PO_4	6.2	2.7–4.5 mg/dL
Sodium	133	135–145 mEq/L
CO_2	18	21–28 mmol/L
Ca^{++}	7.5	8.6–10.0 mg/dL

Abbreviations: ALP, alkaline phosphatase; ALT, alanine aminotransferase; BUN, blood urea nitrogen.

On examination in the laboratory, the CAPD fluid appeared turbid, and the initial Gram's stain revealed many neutrophils and numerous gram-negative bacilli. After overnight incubation, the culture plates (both BAP and chocolate agar) showed large, spreading, gray colonies. Blood cultures showed no growth after 5 days.

Biochemical results from the organism isolated from the CAPD fluid are shown in Table 5–4.

■ Table 5–4 ■ MICROBIOLOGY RESULTS

Dulcitol = negative	Nitrate = positive	Lysine decarboxylase = negative
Sucrose = positive	VP = positive	Arginine dihydrolase = positive
Lactose = positive	Motility = positive	Ornithine decarboxylase = positive
Sorbitol = positive	Indole = negative	Phenylalanine deaminase = negative
Arabinose = positive	DNase = negative	Urea = positive
Citrate = positive	TSI = A/A no H_2S	Oxidase = negative

Abbreviations: VP, Voges-Proskauer; TSI, triple-sugar iron agar.

QUESTIONS

1. Based on the data presented here, what organism is most likely causing Elmer's peritonitis?

2. What general characteristics do members of the family *Enterobacteriaceae* have in common?

3. What biochemical reactions are most helpful when identifying organisms within the family *Enterobacteriaceae*?

4. What biochemical reactions were key to identification of this organism to the genus level?

5. What biochemical reactions were key to identification of this organism to the species level?

6. Many different methods may be used to determine indole production. Independent of the method used for detection, what precursor must be present in the growth media in order to perform an indole test?

7. Explain the nitrate reductase test. Be sure to include the method of detection and the confirmation process.

8. What do the methyl red (MR) and VP tests measure?

9. Given the biochemical reactions of this organism, describe the appearance of this organism on MAC.

10.   a. List the carbohydrates present in TSI and state their relative concentrations.

    b. If an organism is A/A on TSI and colorless on MAC, what can be deduced about that organism with respect to its ability to use each carbohydrate in TSI?

REFERENCES

Carreiro, Eileen. (2000). Personal communication, University of Massachusetts, Dartmouth.

Leclair, Susan J. (2000). Personal communication, University of Massachusetts, Dartmouth.

RECOMMENDED READINGS

Koneman, Elmer W., et al. (1997). *Color Atlas and Textbook of Diagnostic Microbiology.* 5th ed. Philadelphia: J. B. Lippincott.

Mandell, Gerald L., et al. (2000). *Mandell, Douglas, and Bennett's Principles and Practice of Infectious Diseases.* 5th ed., vols. 1 & 2. Philadelphia: Churchill Livingstone.

Murray, Patrick R., et al. (1999). *Manual of Clinical Microbiology.* 7th ed. Washington D.C.: ASM Press.

6 Urinalysis

URINALYSIS CASE 6–1

Karen F., a 40-year-old woman, presented with the following symptoms: flank pain (pain in the side of the trunk between the right or left upper abdomen and the back), fever of 102°F, chills and diaphoresis (sweating), dysuria, nocturia, and increased frequency and urgency of urination. A routine urinalysis was performed (see Table 6–1).

■ Table 6–1 ■ URINALYSIS

	Karen F.	Reference Range
Macroscopic		
Color	Yellow	Colorless to amber
Appearance	Cloudy	Clear
Specific gravity	1.019	1.001–1.035
pH	6.0	5–7
Protein	1+ (30 mg/dL) (SSA:1+)	Neg
Glucose	Neg	Neg
Ketones	Neg	Neg
Bilirubin	Neg	Neg
Blood	1+	Neg
Urobilinogen	Normal	Normal
Nitrite	Pos	Neg
Leukocyte esterase	2+	Neg
Microscopic		
WBCs	40–60/HPF	0–5/HPF
	2–4 clumps/HPF	
RBCs	0–3/HPF	0–2/HPF
Epithelial cells	Few squamous/HPF	Few to moderate
	Rare renal epithelial/HPF	
Casts	3–6 WBC/LPF	Few hyaline
	0–2 granular/LPF	
	0–1 bacterial casts/LPF	
Bacteria	Moderate/HPF	None

Abbreviations: HPF, high-power field; LPF, low-power field; RBCs, red blood cells; SSA, sulfosalicylic acid; WBCs, white blood cells.

QUESTIONS

1. What are the abnormal value(s) or discrepant result(s) in this urinalysis?

2. Are these findings consistent with an upper or lower urinary tract infection (UTI)? Why?

3.   a. Which renal disease/condition is suggested by these urinalysis results?

    b. How would you differentiate acute from chronic?

4. What type of leukocytes are usually associated with pyuria?

5. Which urinalysis finding is pathognomonic (characteristic) of this disease?

6. What are two common physiological causes for this condition?

7. What follow-up test(s) should be ordered, and what would be the most common findings?

8. How is this condition treated?

9. What conditions lead to an increased incidence of this disease—make people more prone to these infections?

10. What is Karen's prognosis?

RECOMMENDED READINGS

Brunzel, Nancy A. (1994). *Fundamentals of Urine and Body Fluid Analysis.* Philadelphia: W. B. Saunders.

Healthanswers. (1999). *Pyelonephritis.* [On-line]. Available: http://www.health answers.com/database/ami/converted/000522.html [1999, February 2].

McBride, Landy J. (1998). *Textbook of Urinalysis and Body Fluids.* Philadelphia: J. B. Lippincott.

Ringsrud, Karen Munson & Jorgenson Linne, Jean. (1995). *Urinalysis and Body Fluids: A Color Text and Atlas.* St. Louis: Mosby.

Strasinger, Susan King. (1994). *Urinalysis and Body Fluids.* Philadelphia: F. A. Davis.

URINALYSIS CASE 6–2

Kate R., a high school basketball player, had been hospitalized with a throat infection, fever, and a question of pneumonia. She had been taking a number of antibiotics. Her physician noted edema and an elevated blood pressure. See Table 6–2.

■ Table 6–2 ■   URINALYSIS AND ADDITIONAL TESTS

| | Urinalysis | |
	Kate R.	Reference Range
Macroscopic		
Color	Red	Colorless to amber
Appearance	Cloudy	Clear
Specific gravity	1.028	1.001–1.035
pH	6.0	5.0–7.0
Protein	2+ (100 mg/dL) (SSA: 2+)	Neg
Glucose	Neg	Neg
Ketones	Neg	Neg
Bilirubin	Neg	Neg
Blood	2+(~50 RBCs/µL)	Neg
Urobilinogen	Normal	Normal
Nitrite	Neg	Neg
Leukocyte esterase	Neg	Neg
Microscopic		
WBCs	0–3/HPF	0–5/HPF
RBCs	30–60/HPF (dysmorphic forms present)	0–2/HPF
Epithelial cells	Few squamous/HPF	Few to moderate
	Rare transitional/HPF	
Casts	1–3 hyaline/LPF	Few hyaline
	0–3 RBC/LPF	
	0–1 hemoglobin/LPF	
	1–3 granular/LPF	
Bacteria	Neg	None

| Additional Urinalysis Tests | | |
	Kate R.	Reference Range
24-h urine volume	400 h	1200–1500 mL/24 h
24-h total protein	1 g/24 h	50–80 mg/24 h

| Chemistry | | |
	Kate R.	Reference Range
BUN	28 mg/dL	7–24 mg/dL
Creatinine	1.6 mg/dL	0.5–1.2 mg/dL

■ **Table 6–2** ■   **URINALYSIS AND ADDITIONAL TESTS** *(continued)*

| | Serology | |
	Kate R.	*Reference Range*
ASO titer	500 TU	< 160TU
Anti-Dnase	Positive	Neg
CH_{50}	60	100–300 CH_{50} units

Abbreviations: ASO, antistreptolysin O; BUN, blood urea nitrogen.

QUESTIONS

1. Circle or highlight the abnormal or discrepant urinalysis result(s).

2. What is the probable diagnosis?

3. Which urinalysis result(s) is/are pathognomic (characteristic) of this condition?

4. Explain the significance of the dysmorphic red cells in the sediment.

5. What is the difference in sensitivity and specificity of the reagent strip protein and the SSA protein?

6. Are the 24-hour urine volume and protein consistent with the diagnosis?

7. What is the probable causative agent (organism) in this case? Briefly describe the pathogenesis (the process).

8. List five other possible causes for this disease.

9. Are the increased BUN and creatinine consistent with the diagnosis?

10. Is the BUN/creatinine ratio consistent with the probable diagnosis?

11. What other renal function test could be performed on the 24-hour urine? Would you expect the results to be decreased, normal, or elevated?

12. Discuss the results of the ASO titer, anti-DNase, and C-3. Are they consistent with the probable diagnosis?

13. What is Kate's prognosis?

RECOMMENDED READINGS

Acute Glomerulonephritis. (1997). [On-line] Available: hhtp://outlinemed.com/demo/nephrol/ [1999, February 2].

Brunzel, Nancy A. (1994). *Fundamentals of Urine and Body Fluid Analysis.* Philadelphia: W. B. Saunders.

McBride, Landy J. (1998). *Textbook of Urinalysis and Body Fluids.* Philadelphia: J. B. Lippincott.

Ringsrud, Karen Munson & Jorgenson Linne, Jean. (1995). *Urinalysis and Body Fluids: A Color Text and Atlas.* St. Louis: Mosby.

Sheehan, Catherine. (1997). *Clinical Immunology: Principles and Laboratory Diagnosis.* Philadelphia: J. B. Lippincott.

Strasinger, Susan King. (1994). *Urinalysis and Body Fluids.* Philadelphia: F. A. Davis.

URINALYSIS CASE 6–3

Bonnie J., a 40-year-old woman with a past history of kidney infections, was seen by her physician because she had felt lethargic for a few weeks. She also complained of decreased frequency of urination and a bloated feeling. The physician noted periorbital swelling and general edema including a swollen abdomen. See Table 6–3.

■ Table 6–3 ■   URINALYSIS AND CHEMISTRY

| | Urinalysis | |
	Bonnie J.	Reference Range
Macroscopic		
Color	Yellow	Colorless to amber
Appearance	Cloudy/Frothy	Clear
Specific gravity	1.022	1.001–1.035
pH	7.0	5–7
Protein	3+ (500 mg/dL) (SSA: 4+)	Neg
Glucose	Neg	Neg
Ketones	Neg	Neg
Bilirubin	Neg	Neg
Blood	Neg	Neg
Urobilinogen	Normal	Normal
Nitrite	Neg	Neg
Leukocyte esterase	Neg	Neg
Microscopic		
WBCs	0–3/HPF	0–5/HPF
RBCs	0–1/HPF	0–2/HPF
Epithelial cells	Rare squamous/HPF	Few to moderate
	Rare renal epithelial/HPF	
Casts	0–3 hyaline/LPF	Few hyaline
	0–1 renal tubular epithelial/LPF	
	0–1 granular/LPF	
	0–1 waxy/LPF	
	0–1 fatty/LPF	
Other	Occasional oval fat bodies	

| | Chemistry | |
	Bonnie J.	Reference Range
Total protein	5.0	6.0–8.4 g/dL
Albumin	2.4	3.5–5.0 g/dL
Cholesterol	370	< 200 mg/dL
BUN	33	7–24 mg/dL
Creatinine	2.1	0.5–1.2 mg/dL

QUESTIONS

1. Circle or highlight the abnormal value(s) or discrepant urinalysis result(s).

2. What type of disease/condition would be characterized by this urinalysis?

3. What is the primary problem/defect found in this condition?

4. What urinalysis result(s) led to your probable diagnosis?

5.   a. What confirmatory test could be performed to identify the oval fat bodies?

b. What is the source of oval fat bodies?

6. Explain the reason for the frothy urine.

7. List five conditions that may progress to this disease (primary or secondary causes of this disease).

8. List five risk factors for this disease.

9. Are the abnormal chemistry tests consistent with the probable diagnosis? Explain why or why not.

10. What other renal function tests could be performed on a 24-hour urine? Would you expect the results to be decreased, normal, or elevated?

11. Discuss the physiological cause of the edema.

12. Describe what you would expect to see in Bonnie's protein electrophoresis.

13. What is the protein selectivity index? What can it tell the physician about the type of renal damage?

14. What are some of the possible consequences (complications) of this condition—what could it lead to?

REFERENCES

Brunzel, Nancy A. (1994). *Fundamentals of Urine and Body Fluid Analysis.* Philadelphia: W. B. Saunders.

Burtis, Carl A. & Ashwood, Edward R. (1996). *Tietz Fundamentals of Clinical Chemistry.* 4th ed. Philadelphia: W. B. Saunders.

McBride, Landy J. (1998). *Textbook of Urinalysis and Body Fluids.* Philadelphia: J. B. Lippincott.

Ringsrud, Karen Munson & Jorgenson Linne, Jean. (1995). *Urinalysis and Body Fluids: A Color Text and Atlas.* St. Louis: Mosby.

RxMed. (1999). *Nephrotic Syndrome.* [On-line] Available: http://www.rxmed.com/ illnesses/nephrotic_syndrome.html [1999, February 8].

Strasinger, Susan King. (1994). *Urinalysis and Body Fluids.* Philadelphia: F. A. Davis.

URINALYSIS CASE 6–4

Andrea R., a 22-two-year-old MLT student, performed a macroscopic urinalysis on her own urine as part of the macroscopic urinalysis laboratory. She noted some dysuria, frequency, and urgency of urination. The program director recommended that Andrea contact her physician for a complete routine urinalysis and possible culture and sensitivity. See Table 6–4.

■ Table 6–4 ■   URINALYSIS

| | Andrea R. | | |
	Day1*	Day 2*	Reference Range
Macroscopic			
Color	Yellow	Yellow	Colorless to amber
Appearance	Cloudy	Cloudy	Clear
Specific gravity	1.013	1.016	1.001–1.035
pH	7.0	7.5	5–7
Protein	Neg	Neg	Neg
Glucose	Neg	Neg	Neg
Ketones	Neg	Neg	Neg
Bilirubin	Neg	Neg	Neg
Blood	Neg	Neg	Neg
Urobilinogen	Normal	Normal	Normal
Nitrite	Positive	Positive	Neg
Leukocyte esterase	2+	2+	Neg
Microscopic			
WBCs	NT	25–40/HPF	0–5/HPF
RBCs	NT	0–3/HPF	0–2/HPF
Epithelial cells	NT	Few squamous/HPF	Few to moderate
		Few transitional/HPF	
Casts	NT	Neg	Few hyaline
Bacteria	NT	Moderate	Negative

*Day 1, macroscopic performed at school; day 2, performed on physician's order.
Abbreviation: NT, not tested.

QUESTIONS

1. Circle or highlight the abnormal or discrepant urinalysis result(s).

2.   a. Do the abnormal results indicate an upper or lower urinary tract infection?

b. What single finding is most helpful in determining the source of the infection? Why?

3. What is the probable disease/condition?

4. Would you change your answer if either the leukocyte esterase or nitrite were negative and the microscopic remained the same? Explain why or why not.

5. Explain the presence of increased transitional epithelial cells in this condition.

6. What bacteria are most commonly identified in this condition?

7. What fruit juice is often recommended to reduce pyuria and bacteruria?

8. Why are patients instructed to increase their fluid intake?

9. Why are women more prone to this condition than men?

10. What conditions are associated with an increased incidence of this infection?

RECOMMENDED READING

Brunzel, Nancy A. (1994). *Fundamentals of Urine and Body Fluid Analysis.* Philadelphia: W. B. Saunders.

Graber, Mark A. & Martinez-Bianchi, Viviana. (1999). *Genitourinary and Renal Disease: Urinary Tract Infections: Females.* [On-line] Available: http://www.vh.org/Providers/ClinRef/FPHandbook/Chapter11/01-11.html [1999, March 10].

McBride, Landy J. (1998). *Textbook of Urinalysis and Body Fluids.* Philadelphia: J. B. Lippincott.

Ringsrud, Karen Munson & Jorgenson Linne, Jean. (1995). *Urinalysis and Body Fluids: A Color Text and Atlas.* St. Louis: Mosby.

Strasinger, Susan King. (1994). *Urinalysis and Body Fluids.* Philadelphia: F. A. Davis.

URINALYSIS CASE 6–5

Sean F., a 25-year-old man, was brought to the emergency room with severe crush injuries sustained in a car accident. He had a broken pelvis and right femur and numerous abrasions and contusions. A routine urinalysis was ordered as part of the regular preoperative bloodwork (see Table 6–5).

■ Table 6–5 ■   URINALYSIS AND CHEMISTRY

	Urinalysis	
	Sean F.	Reference Range
Macroscopic		
Color	Brown	Colorless to amber
Appearance	Clear	Clear
Specific gravity	1.013	1.001–1.035
pH	6.0	5–7
Protein	1+	Neg
Glucose	Neg	Neg
Ketones	Neg	Neg
Bilirubin	Neg	Neg
Blood	3+	Neg
Urobilinogen	Normal	Normal
Nitrite	Neg	Neg
Leukocyte esterase	Neg	Neg
Microscopic		
WBCs	0–3/HPF	0–5/HPF
RBCs	0–1/HPF	0–2/HPF
Epithelial cells	Few squamous/HPF	Few to moderate
	Few renal epithelial/HPF	
Casts	0–2 hyaline/LPF	Few hyaline
	0–1 granular/LPF	
Bacteria	Neg	None
	Chemistry	
	Sean F.	Reference Range
Creatine kinase	170,000 IU/L	24–170 IU/L
Lactate dehydrogenase	2,500 IU/L	91–192 IU/L

QUESTIONS

1. Circle or highlight abnormal or discrepant urinalysis and chemistry result(s).

2. What two substances can give a positive reagent strip for blood and a negative microscopic finding?

3. List five causes for each of these two conditions (substances in question 2).

4. What is the most probable explanation for the positive blood reagent strip reaction?

5. Briefly explain the pathophysiology (what happens) in this disease/condition.

6. Describe the confirmatory test(s) for the condition in question 4.

7. How would you explain the presence of casts and renal epithelial cells?

8. Why are the creatine kinase and lactate dehydrogenase elevated?

9. What additional lab tests would be helpful?

RECOMMENDED READINGS

Brunzel, Nancy A. (1994). *Fundamentals of Urine and Body Fluid Analysis.* Philadelphia: W. B. Saunders.

Burtis, Carl A. & Ashwood, Edward R. (1999). *Tietz Textbook of Clinical Chemistry.* 3rd ed. Philadelphia: W. B. Saunders.

Dhawan, Rajiv, Jyothinagaran, Madhu G. & Shwartz, Allan B. (1999). *Pathogenesis and Management of Rhabdomyolysis.* [On-line] Available: www.auhs.edu/continuing/cme/medicine/pathogen/introduc.htm [1999, March 3].

McBride, Landy J. (1998). *Textbook of Urinalysis and Body Fluids.* Philadelphia: J. B. Lippincott.

Ringsrud, Karen Munson & Jorgenson Linne, Jean. (1995). *Urinalysis and Body Fluids: A Color Text and Atlas.* St. Louis: Mosby.

Strasinger, Susan King. (1994). *Urinalysis and Body Fluids.* Philadelphia: F. A. Davis.

URINALYSIS CASE 6–6

Tammy S., a 20-year-old long-distance runner, went to the University Health Center for her physical following the first practice of the season. The results of her urinalysis are shown in Table 6–6.

■ Table 6–6 ■ URINALYSIS

	Tammy S.	Reference Range
Macroscopic		
Color	Amber	Colorless to amber
Appearance	Clear	Clear
Specific gravity	1.028	1.001–1.035
pH	7.0	5–7
Protein	Trace 5–20 mg/dL (SSA: trace)	Neg
Glucose	Neg	Neg
Ketones	Neg	Neg
Bilirubin	Neg	Neg
Blood	1+	Neg
Urobilinogen	4 mg/dL	Normal
Nitrite	Neg	Neg
Leukocyte esterase	Trace	Neg
Microscopic		
WBCs	10–20/HPF	0–5/HPF
RBCs	30–40/HPF	0–2/HPF
Epithelial cells	Few squamous/HPF	Few to moderate
Casts	10–20 hyaline/LPF	Few hyaline
	10–15 granular/LPF	
Bacteria	Neg	None
Crystals	Neg	

QUESTIONS

1. What are the abnormal or discrepant urinalysis results?

2. List five possible explanations for these abnormal results.

3. Should Tammy be concerned about these results?

4. What is the most likely explanation for the abnormal results?

5. What is the usual source of granular casts in pathological conditions, e.g., glomerulonephritis?

6. What would the physician do to follow up on this athlete?

7.   a. How could you differentiate granular casts from pathological condi-
        tions and those formed in nonpathological conditions?

      b. What clues are in the urinalysis report?

RECOMMENDED READINGS

Brunzel, Nancy A. (1994). *Fundamentals of Urine and Body Fluid Analysis.* Philadelphia: W. B. Saunders.

McBride, Landy J. (1998). *Textbook of Urinalysis and Body Fluids.* Philadelphia: J. B. Lippincott.

Ringsrud, Karen Munson & Jorgenson Linne, Jean. (1995). *Urinalysis and Body Fluids: A Color Text and Atlas.* St. Louis: Mosby.

Strasinger, Susan King. (1994). *Urinalysis and Body Fluids.* Philadelphia: F. A. Davis.

URINALYSIS CASE 6–7

A medical technologist reviewed the urinalysis report shown in Table 6–7 before it was released to the physician.

■ Table 6–7 ■   URINALYSIS

	Patient	Reference Range
Macroscopic		
Color	Yellow	Colorless to amber
Appearance	Slightly Cloudy	Clear
Specific gravity	1.015	1.001–1.035
pH	7.0	5–7
Protein	Neg	Neg
Glucose	Neg	Neg
Ketones	Neg	Neg
Bilirubin	Neg	Neg
Blood	Neg	Neg
Urobilinogen	Normal	Normal
Nitrite	Neg	Neg
Leukocyte esterase	Neg	Neg
Microscopic		
WBCs	0–1/HPF	0–5/HPF
RBCs	25–30/HPF	0–2/HPF
Epithelial cells	Rare squamous/HPF	Few to moderate
Casts	Neg	Few hyaline
Bacteria	Neg	None

QUESTIONS

1. What urinalysis results are abnormal or discrepant?

2. What is the technologist's first course of action to investigate the results?

3. What should the technologist do next?

4. What are five possible explanations for these results?

5. List five structures that can be confused with RBCs.

6. How would you differentiate the confusing structures from RBCs?

7. How would you rule out the other possible explanations in question 4?

RECOMMENDED READINGS

Brunzel, Nancy A. (1994). *Fundamentals of Urine and Body Fluid Analysis.* Philadelphia: W. B. Saunders.

McBride, Landy J. (1998). *Textbook of Urinalysis and Body Fluids.* Philadelphia: J. B. Lippincott.

Ringsrud, Karen Munson & Jorgenson Linne, Jean. (1995). *Urinalysis and Body Fluids: A Color Text and Atlas.* St. Louis: Mosby.

Strasinger, Susan King. (1994). *Urinalysis and Body Fluids.* Philadelphia: F. A. Davis.

Answers to Chapter Cases

BLOOD BANK CASE 1–1 ANSWERS

1. Paul's forward grouping is AB, and the reverse grouping is A. He is probably A Rh_o (D)-positive.

2. The discrepant result is the 1+ reaction with anti-B in the forward grouping. The reaction with anti-B is much weaker (1+) than with anti-A (4+).

3. This is a case of acquired B phenotype. Acquired B antigens are usually associated with the presence of intestinal bacteria in the blood stream from intestinal obstruction, carcinoma of the colon or rectum, and other lower intestinal tract disorders. Two processes have been described that can result in acquired B. The first and most common is the bacterial enzymatic effect on the A receptors in group A_1 individuals. Bacterial deacetylating enzymes modify the group A immunodominant sugar, N-acetyl-D-galactosamine, into D-galactoseamine, which will cross react with anti-B antisera. The second is the increased permeability of the intestinal wall, which leads to the absorption of the B-like bacterial polysaccharides onto cells, causing B specificity in group A or O individuals.

4. *Escherichia coli* O_{86} and *Proteus vulgaris* are two bacteria commonly associated with acquired B.

5. The technologist should

   a. Check patient diagnosis. Is it consistent with acquired B? Does the patient have a gastrointestinal problem?

   b. Test the patient's serum against autologous red cells. The patient's anti-B will not agglutinate his or her red blood cells (RBCs) with the acquired B antigen.

   c. Test the patient's RBCs with monoclonal anti-B reagent. The non-human monoclonal antibodies will not react with acquired B antigen. Check the package insert carefully to verify this is the case with the monoclonal antiserum used (some may react with acquired B).

   d. Test the patient's RBCs with human anti-B that has been acidified to pH 6.0. Acquired B will not react with anti-B at pH 6.0.

   e. Treat the patient's RBCs with acetic anhydride, which will reacetylate the A and diminish the strength of the acquired B. Normal group B will not be affected by acetic anhydride.

6. Yes, the negative antibody screen rules out the common alloantibodies and autoantibodies.

7.   a. Secretors can produce glycoproteins, e.g., H, in their epithelial secretions including saliva. They can secrete H, which can be converted to A and/or B if the person carries the A and/or B gene.

   b. They comprise about 80% of the population.

   c. Paul's secretions would contain H and A antigens. He does not have the B gene, therefore B would not be found in his secretions.

8. Acquired B will disappear once the condition that caused it is cured or under control.

BLOOD BANK CASE 1–2 ANSWERS

1. Lisa is A Rh_o (D)-positive.

2. The antibody screen is positive, indicating an unexpected antibody in the patient's serum.

3. The antibody is most likely immunoglobulin G (IgG) because the immediate spin (IS) is negative and the strongest phase of reaction was antihuman globulin (AHG).

4. It is an alloantibody. Autoantibody can be ruled out on the basis of the negative autocontrol.

5. Lisa has had a previous pregnancy (second child); therefore she could have been sensitized with her first baby. We do not know if she has ever been transfused, but the first pregnancy is a likely source of stimulation for the alloantibody.

6. The next step would be an antibody panel to identify the antibody detected by the antibody screen.

7. Antibodies are ruled out using the rule-out cells. Rule-out cells are the panel cells that are negative in *all* phases at which the panel was tested. Using the rule-out cells, the technician can rule out antibodies when cells homozygous for the antigen do not react with the antibody, because if the antibody was present, it would have reacted with the antigen on the cell. Therefore, all antibodies in the rule-out cells that are homozygous positive for the antigen can be ruled out. Panel procedures vary from institution to institution; some laboratories eliminate all antibodies when cells are positive for the antigen and do *not* react with the antibody in the patient's serum whether or not the cell is homozygous or heterozygous. In the majority of cases, this will not cause a problem and it will usually work very well with routine single antibodies that do not exhibit dosage.

8. Only antibodies that are negative with homozygous cells can be ruled out, because antibodies such as anti-M, anti-N, anti-S, anti-s, anti-C, anti-E, anti-c, anti-e, anti-Fy^a, anti-Fy^b, anti-Jk^a, and anti-Jk^b may show dosage. They may react weakly or not at all with heterozygous cells.

9. Anti-E, anti-c, anti-f, anti-V, anti-M, anti-N, anti-Lu^a, anti-K, anti-Js^a, and anti-Fy^a cannot be ruled out. Anti-M, anti-N, anti-K, and anti-Fy^a were not ruled out, because the cells were heterozygous.

10. The most likely antibody is anti-c, because the pattern of reactions with the patient's serum matches exactly the c antigen reaction column (positive with cells 1 to 6, 10, and 11; negative with cells 7 to 9).

11. a. The 3 + 3 rule states that at least three cells in the panel are *positive* for the antigen and react with the antibody and at least three cells in the panel are *negative* for the antigen and do not react with the antibody. The 3 + 3 rule gives a probability value (P) of .05 or less to call the results valid. A P value of 0.05 indicates a 5% or less chance of these results occurring randomly; in other words, a 95% or greater chance of having correctly identified the antibody(ies).

    b. Thus, anti-c meets the 3 + 3 rule.

12. a. Lisa's Fisher-Race phenotype is D_CCEe.

    b. The antigen phenotype provides additional evidence to confirm anti-c and to rule out anti-E. Lisa is negative for c (homozygous CC); therefore, anti-c alloantibody is possible. She is positive for E and K, which rules out anti-E and anti-K alloantibodies. Anti-f can also be ruled out, since Lisa is c negative. (If the patient is c negative or e negative, he or she is f negative; f is only present when c and e are inherited as a haplotype.)

13. The screening cell antigram does not rule out anti-E, anti-c, anti-f, anti-V, anti-M, anti-N, anti-s, anti-Le^a, anti-Lu^a, anti-K, anti-k, anti-Kp^a, anti-Js^a, anti-Fy^a, and anti-Jk^b. The screening antigram supports the identification of anti-c.

14. Additional cells that can be set up:

    a. 2 cells: c negative, V positive (to meet 3+3 rule)

    b. 1 cell: c negative, M positive, N negative

    c. 1 cell: c negative, N positive, M negative

    d. 1 cell: c negative, Js^a positive

    e. c negative, Fy^a positive, Fy^b negative

    These five cells should be negative with the patient's serum if anti-c is the only antibody. If they are negative, the antibodies are ruled out. Lu^a is usually not clinically significant.

15. The units selected for crossmatch must be c negative, so antigen typing for c-negative units is added to the crossmatch procedure.

BLOOD BANK CASE # 3 ANSWERS

1. Jim is O Rh₀ (D)-positive.

2. The antibody screen is positive, indicating the presence of an unexpected antibody.

3. The antibody(ies) is/are most likely IgG. IgG antibodies usually do not react on IS (room temperature), and their strongest reactions are at AHG.

4. Anti-E, anti-Lu^a, anti-K, anti-Kp^a, and anti-Js^a cannot be ruled out.

5. No, none of the antibodies is a perfect match for the panel results.

6. Some possible explanations:
   a. Multiple antibodies are present.
   b. One of the antibodies exhibits dosage. This can be eliminated because of the use of only homozygous cells for ruling out antibodies.
   c. Variations unrelated to zygosity. Some antigens (I, P_1, Lewis, and Sd^a) vary in strength among individuals whether they are homozygous or heterozygous.
   d. Antibodies against high-frequency or low-frequency antigens.
   e. Cold-reactive autoantibodies. These can be eliminated as possibilities because of the negative reaction at IS.
7. The most likely explanation is multiple antibodies. Although all of the positive cells react at the same phases (37 and AHG), there is some variability in strength of reaction(s) (1+-3+).
8. The most likely antibodies are anti-E and anti-K. Cells 4 and 10 are positive for E, and cells 2, 8, and 11 are positive for K. Panel results are cells 2, 4, 8, 10, and 11 positive and the remaining cells negative.
9. Three procedures to confirm antibody identification are
   a. Phenotype the patient's cells for the corresponding antigen. (Antigen typing the patient's cell to determine which antigens are present.) The antigen should *not* be present on the patient's red cells; in other words, if the patient has the antibody, the patient's cells should be negative for the antigen.
   b. Review the screening cell antigram. Does the antigram confirm or dispute the suspected antibody(ies)? Are the three screening cells positive in the cells that test positive for E and K and negative in any cells that are negative for both antigens?
   c. Type prospective donor units to find antigen negative units for crossmatch. If a unit negative for the antigen(s) comes up incompatible in crossmatch, an error was made in identification of the antibody. Either the antibody was incorrectly identified, or another antibody is present that was not identified.
10. a. Jim's Rh and Kell phenotypes do not rule out anti-E or anti-K. He is negative for both antigens; therefore, alloantibodies to these two antigens are possible.
    b. The screening cell antigram helps to confirm anti-E and anti-K. Cell II is positive for E and cell I is positive for K, and the patient's serum reacted with both. Cell III is negative for both, and the patient was negative in cell III. Anti-D, anti-C, anti-E, anti-C^w, anti-V, anti-M, anti-S, anti-Le^b, anti-Lu^a, anti-K, anti-Kp^a, anti-Js^a, anti-Fy^b, and anti-Jk^a are not ruled out by the antibody screen. Of those not eliminated by the antibody screen, anti-D, anti-C, anti-C^w, anti-V, anti-M, anti-S, anti-Le^b, anti-Fy^b, and anti-Jk^a were eliminated by the antibody panel. No results are given to evaluate this confirmatory procedure.

11. Anti-Lu^a, anti-Kp^a, and anti-Js^a can be ruled out because of their low frequency and clinical insignificance.

12. The donor units must be phenotyped and the patient crossmatched with units negative for E and K antigens.

13. a. To determine the percentage of units that would be compatible, the percentage of the population (donors) negative for the first antigen is multiplied by the percentage of the population negative for the second antigen and so on. In this case, 91% of the population are K negative and 70% are E negative; therefore, $0.91 \times 0.70 = 0.64$. Therefore, 64% of the population would be negative for both.

   b. To determine approximately how many units we would have to test to find five compatible units, we would determine 64% of what (x) would equal 5 (simple algebra)

$$0.64 \times x = 5 \qquad x = \frac{5}{.64} x = 8$$

Sixty-four percent of units are compatible (E and K antigen negative); therefore, 7.8 U or 8 U, are needed to find five K-negative and E-negative units.

BLOOD BANK CASE 1–4 ANSWERS

1. Ruth is type A Rh$_o$ (D)-positive.

2. The antibody screen is positive, indicating the presence of an unexpected antibody(ies).

3. Ruth's autocontrol is negative, ruling out the presence of autoantibodies. The variability in the strength of reactions (3+ and ±) points toward the presence of multiple alloantibodies.

4. In Figure 1–3, anti-C^w, anti-V, anti-K, anti-Fy^a, anti-Jk^a, anti-Le^b, anti-N, and anti-Lu^a cannot be ruled out using cells that are homozygous for the antigen. Anti-K, anti-Fy^a, and anti-Jk^a could have been ruled out using cell 7, but it is *heterozygous* for K, Fy^a and Jk^a.

5. The screening cell antigram cannot rule out anti-D, anti-C, anti-E, anti-c, anti-V, anti-K, anti-k, anti-Kp^b, anti-Js^b, anti-Fy^a, anti-Fy^b, anti-Jk^a, anti-Jk^b, anti-Le^a, anti-s, anti-N, anti-P$_1$, and anti-Lu^a.

6. The screening cell antigram does rule out anti-C^w and anti-Le^b, which are not eliminated by Figure 1–3. Anti-D, anti-C, anti-E, anti-c, anti-k, anti-Kp^b, anti-Js^b, anti-Fy^b, anti-Jk^b, anti-Le^a, anti-s, and anti-P$_1$ are ruled out by Figure 1–3.

7. Anti-E, anti-C^w, anti-V, anti-K, anti-Kp^a, anti-Js^a, anti-Fy^a, anti-Jk^a, anti-s, anti-N, and anti-Lu^a are not ruled out in Figure 1–4 using only cells homozygous for the antigens.

8. If the results of Figures 1–3 and 1–4 and the antibody screen are combined, then anti-E, anti-Kp^a, anti-Js^a, and anti-s are ruled out in Figure 1–3. The screening cell antigram rules out anti-C^w and anti-Le^b.

Figure 1–3	Antibody Screen	Figure 1–4
anti-C^w	anti-D	anti-E
anti-V	anti-C	anti-C^w
anti-K	anti-E	**anti-V**
anti-Fy^a	anti-c	**anti-K**
anti-Jk^a	**anti-V**	anti-Kp^a
anti-Le^b	**anti-K**	anti-Js^a
anti-N	anti-k	**anti-Fy^a**
anti-Lu^a	anti-Kp^b	**anti-Jk^a**
	anti-Js^b	anti-s
	anti-Fy^a	**anti-N**
	anti-Fy^b	**anti-Lu^a**
	anti- Jk^a	
	anti-Jk^b	
	anti-Le^a	
	anti-s	
	anti-N	
	anti-P_1	
	anti-Lu^a	

The remaining antibodies are those that are common to all three lists; in other words, they were not ruled out by either of the two panels or the antibody screen. These are anti-V, anti-K, anti-Jk^a, anti-Fy^a, anti-N, and anti-Lu^a.

9. Ruth has anti-K and anti-Jk^a. It is important to note that cells 3 and 4 on Figure 1–4 are heterozygous for Jk^a and react very weakly due to dosage!

10. The antigen typing supports the antibody identification. Ruth is negative for the antigens. Anti-Fy^a is eliminated because she is positive for the antigen.

BLOOD BANK CASE 1–5 ANSWERS

1. Mary is A Rh_o (D)-positive.

2. Mary has an alloantibody(ies). Autoantibodies can be ruled out by the negative autocontrol.

3. The screening cell antigram cannot rule out anti-C, anti-e, anti-f, anti-C^w, anti-V, anti-K, anti-Kp^a, anti-Js^a, anti-Fy^a, anti-Jk^b, anti-Xg^a, anti-Le^a, anti-S, anti-s, anti-M, and anti Lu^a. Anti-f can be ruled out because the cell is negative for e. (f is present only when c and e are inherited as a haplotypeon the same chromosome.)

4. Figure 1–5 cannot rule out anti-E, anti-C^w, anti-K, anti-Kp^a, anti-Js^a, anti-Fy^a, anti-Jk^b, anti-Le^a, anti-N, and anti Lu^a.

5. The following antibodies cannot be ruled out by either the antibody screen or Figure 1–5: anti-C^w, anti-K, anti-Kp^a, anti-Js^a, anti-Fy^a, anti-Jk^b, anti-Le^a, anti Lu^a. *Note:* Anti-C, anti-e, anti-f, anti-V, anti-Xg^a, anti-S, anti-s, and anti-M are ruled out by Figure 1–5; anti-E and anti-N are ruled out by the screening cell antigram.

6. Ficin or papain inactivate the following antigens, therefore the antibodies would not react with enzyme-treated cells: M, N, S, Fy^a, Fy^b, Fy6, Yt^a, Ch, Rg, Pr, Xg^a, JMH, Ge2. Ficin or papain enhances the reactivity of the following antigens, Rh, Kidd, Lewis, and some Kell. Therefore some antibodies will have stronger reactions with enzyme-treated cells.

7. Polyethylene glycol (PEG) increases the sensitivity by concentrating a weak antibody in a low ionic strength environment (LISS), which enhances the rate of antibody uptake. It removes water molecules, bringing sensitized RBCs closer together to increase the likelihood of antigen–antibody binding and agglutination. It can be used only with monospecific anti-IgG AHG.

8. The antibody identified by the enzyme-pretreated panel (Figure 1–6) is anti-K. The panel reactions match anti-K exactly and are 2+ or 3+. The antibodies that cannot be ruled out are anti-Kp^a, anti-Js^a, and anti-Lu^a.

9. The antibodies identified by the ImmuAdd and PEG Figure 1–6 are anti-K and anti-Fy^a. Anti-E was ruled out by antibody screen. Anti-C^w, anti-Kp^a, anti-Js^a, anti-Le^a, and anti Lu^a cannot be ruled out.

10. Mary's probable genotype is R_2R_2 (DcE/DcE).

11. The antigen typing supports the identification of anti-K and anti-Fy^a. The patient is negative for those antigens and positive for Fy^b.

12. Ninety-one percent of the population is K negative, and 34% is Fy^a negative. K (0.91) × Fy^a (0.34) = 30.9% = 31% of donors should be compatible. 0.31 × (number of units) = 3. Number of units = ~ 9.7 = 10 U. Approximately 31% of donors would be negative for both K and Fy^a; therefore 10 U should yield 3 compatible units (K-, Fy^a-). You can also use the following formula:

$$\frac{\text{No. of units needed}}{\text{\% of population without the antigens}} = \text{No. of units to be tested}$$

$$\frac{3}{(0.91) \times (0.34)} = 10 \text{ U would have to be tested to find 3 U negative for Kell and Fy}^a$$

BLOOD BANK CASE 1–6 ANSWERS

1. The initial antibody screen (11/21/00) is negative; therefore, Jane does not have any detectable alloantibodies at this point.

2. The most likely explanation for a drop in hemoglobin and hematocrit following a transfusion is a hemolytic process, although hemorrhaging must be ruled out.

3. The postoperative antibody screen is positive for an alloantibody(ies). Screening cell 1 is positive as well as the autocontrol.

4. The positive autocontrol indicates that antibody and/or complement is coating RBCs. Usually, the patient has a positive direct antiglobulin test and/or an autoantibody. Positive autocontrols are associated with hemolytic transfusion reactions, autoimmune hemolytic anemias, and drug-induced hemolytic anemias.

5. a. The direct antiglobulin test is positive with polyspecific antihuman globulin (AHG) and monospecific anti-IgG and negative with anticomplement. This provides further evidence of an alloantibody in the patient's serum reacting with an antigen on recently transfused donor RBCs.

   b. The technologist would run an antibody panel on Jane's serum to identify the alloantibody(ies).

6. The following antibodies cannot be ruled out by the antibody panel in Figure 1–8: anti-E, anti-C^w, anti-V, anti-K, anti-Kp^a, anti-Js^a, anti-Fy^a, anti-Jk^b, anti-S, anti-Lu^a.

7. The difference in strength of reaction can be explained by dosage. Cells 1, 2, and 8 with 3+ reactions are homozygous for Jk^b, and cells 3, 4, 9, and 10 with 2+ reactions are heterozygous for Jk^b.

8. The most likely antibody (because it matches the antigram perfectly) is anti-Jk^b.

9. The remaining antibodies can be ruled out using a panel of cells that are Jk^b negative and homozygous for E, K, Js^a, and S. C^w, V, Kp^a, and Lu^a are low-incidence antigens and are not clinically significant under normal circumstances. They should not cause problems with crossmatching.

10. The eluate reactions do confirm anti-Jk^b, identified in question 6. The Jk^b heterozygous cells (cells 3, 4, 9, and 10) are weak, and the Jk^b homozygous cells (cells 1, 2, and 8) are 1+.

11. Jane is a classic case of delayed hemolytic transfusion reaction (DHTR) caused by an anamnestic response 7 to 14 days post-transfusion. The original antibody screen on 1/22 was negative, due to undetectable levels of anti-Jk^b. She had been sensitized by the original transfusion, and the transfusion of Jk^b-positive donor cells stimulated the production of IgG anti-Jk^b by the memory cells. This process takes a few days, hence a DHTR. Other antibodies associated with DHTR are anti-E, anti-D, anti-C, anti-K, anti-Fy^a, and anti-M. A fall in hemoglobin and hematocrit following a transfusion should be investigated as a possible DHTR.

12. Review of transfusion history is critical in any transfusion workup in preventing DHTRs due to antibodies that may have decreased to undetectable levels. Kidd antibodies are notorious for being difficult to detect, exhibiting dosage as in this case, and causing DHTRs.

13. Serum bilirubin (total and direct), hemoglobin, haptoglobin, urine bilirubin, urine hemoglobin, and urobilinogen. Serum bilirubin (total and indirect) is usually elevated by the hemolysis of donor erythrocytes. Hemoglobinemia and hemoglobinuria are not usually present in DHTR. Haptoglobin is a mucoprotein that binds to free hemoglobin in the plasma.

It is decreased in hemolytic transfusion reactions because it is used faster than the liver can produce it. Coagulation studies (prothrombin time and activated partial thromboplastin time) and renal function tests (blood urea nitrogen and creatinine) may be ordered to monitor for disseminated intravascular coagulation and renal failure, which are rare complications of DHTR.

BLOOD BANK CASE 1–7 ANSWERS

1. The increased bilirubin was most likely caused by hemolysis of the baby's RBCs by maternal antibodies or hemolytic disease of the newborn (HDN). HDN occurs when the baby inherits an antigen from the father—in this case, A_1—which the mother does not have. The mother produces antibodies against the antigen, but in this case, anti-A_1 is non-red cell stimulated and is already present in the mother's serum.

2. The genotype is the total genetic makeup: the pair of genes that were inherited from the parents, one from the father and one from the mother. The genotype is always indicated as two alleles, for example, AA, which means the individual inherited the A allele from both parents. The phenotype is the genes expressed by the individual, the observable traits. In this case, ABO and Rh antigens are detected. For example, without family studies it is impossible to determine whether a B individual is BB or BO.

3. The mother's ABO genotype is OO, and her Rh (D) genotype is Dd. (She is Rh positive, but the baby inherited d from both parents.) There is no d allele, but d is sometimes used to indicate the absence of D. The baby's ABO phenotype is A_1 (which she could have inherited from either parent), and her Rh is dd. She inherited d from both parents.

4. No, routine prenatal testing would not have helped to predict this HDN. No specific tests can be performed that could predict the possibility of ABO HDN.

5. Reverse grouping is not performed on newborns, because ABO antibodies are not produced. If a reverse grouping were done, it would detect maternal antibodies.

6. HDN is categorized in three categories by antibody specificity:
   a. Rh HDN
   b. ABO HDN
   c. Other (Non-Rh) antibodies

7. This case is categorized as an ABO HDN because of the anti-A_1 found in the eluate. ABO can affect first pregnancies because ABO antibodies are naturally occurring (non-red cell stimulated) in the mother's serum.

8. ABO HDN with group O mothers and group A babies is the most common scenario because of the high-titered IgG antibodies in group O individuals. Therefore, group O mothers with potent anti-A,B are the mostly likely candidates for babies with ABO HDN.

9. The anti-A$_1$ is IgG because it passed through the placenta. IgG is the only immunoglobulin class that can pass from the mother to the fetus. IgG is transported across the placenta from the second trimester until the baby is born.

10. Elution testing is performed using antihuman globulin because the antibody of interest is IgG. IgG, which can cross the placenta (see question 9), reacts best in the presence of antihuman globulin.

11. A fetal screen/Kleihauer-Betke is not required in this case. The incompatibility is not Rh(D); therefore, neither a fetal screen/Kleihauer-Betke nor Rhogam is required. These are only used in cases of Rh(D) HDN.

12. The physician would monitor the baby's hemoglobin, hematocrit, and bilirubin for signs of increased hemolysis.

13. Jaundice in ABO HDN is usually mild and can be treated with phototherapy if indicated. The anemia is usually mild and will resolve itself. Severe anemia requiring exchange transfusion is very rare in ABO HDN.

14. No, there is no way to prevent this from happening in future pregnancies. ABO HDN can occur in the first pregnancy or in following pregnancies, or it may not occur at all. There is no way of predicting the possibility of an ABO HDN.

15. No, cord bloods should be saved in the blood bank but only tested if the physician suspects HDN.

BLOOD BANK CASE 1–8 ANSWERS

Patient 1

1. Yes, Anne's hemoglobin is close to the critical level of 6 g/dL for surgical and leukemic patients, even though, she is *not* having surgery. She is symptomatic, and the anemia is definitely affecting her quality of life.

2. No, there are no absolutes in transfusion therapy for a patient who is not actively hemorrhaging. Anne could take iron supplements and have her hemoglobin and hematocrit monitored regularly. The physician and patient should discuss the pros and cons of transfusion and alternative therapy, and the patient should be allowed to make the correct decision in her case. Of course, treating the cause of the anemia should be a primary concern.

3. The results of her complete blood count (CBC) and medical history indicate an iron-deficiency anemia, hypochromic and microcytic.

4. Anne needs the oxygen-carrying capacity of RBCs to relieve her symptoms, indicating packed RBCs would be the component of choice. To raise her hemoglobin to 10 g/dL, she would need a minimum of 3 U ($1.5 \times 3 = 4.5$ g/dL).

5.
   a. Each unit of packed RBCs will raise the hemoglobin of a 70-kg man 1 to 1.5 g/dL; therefore, 3 U should raise her hemoglobin by at least 3 g/dL, from 6.1 g/dL to 9.1 g/dL. The maximum would be 1.5 g/dL $\times$ 3 = 4.5 g/dL + 6.1 = 10.6 g/dL.

b. In the case of smaller individuals (< 155 lbs/70 kg), the increase should be slightly greater.

Patient 2

6. Yes, a platelet count of 19,000/μL would indicate a need for platelet transfusion before surgery. A platelet count under 20,000/μL is usually the criterion for prophylactic platelet transfusion, especially for a surgical patient.

7. Each unit of platelets will raise the platelet count by 5,000 to 10,000/μL in a 70-kg man. A platelet count of 50,000/μL is considered minimal for an invasive procedure; therefore, 4 U of platelets should be administered (7,500/μL × 4 = 30,000/μL).

8. Carl's platelet count 1 hour post-transfusion should be at least 50,000/μL.

9.   a. The corrected count increment (CCI) is

$$\frac{\text{Post-TPC} - \text{Pre-TPC}}{\text{No. platelets transfused}} \times \text{BSA}$$

Where BSA is body surface area, Post-TPC is post-transfusion platelet count; Pre-TPC is pretransfusion platelet count. Therefore,

$$\frac{42,000\text{-}\mu L - 19,000/\mu L}{4 \times 0.55/U} \times 1.5 \text{ m}^2 = \frac{23,000}{2.2} = 10,545/\mu L$$

    b. A CCI over 10,000 indicates an adequate response to platelet transfusion: The patient is benefiting from the transfusion, and the platelets are surviving.

    c. In other words, the patient is *not* refractory to platelets.

10. Platelets are stored at room temperature (20 to 24°C) with constant agitation and have a shelf-life of 5 days in a closed system. If the seal is broken, the shelf-life is reduced to 4 hours.

Patient 3

11. Melissa's results would most likely be

    a. Prothrombin time: Normal

    b. Activated partial thromboplastin time: Increased

    c. Platelet count: Normal

    d. Bleeding time: Increased

    e. VIII:C: Decreased

    f. Ristocetin-induced platelet aggregation: Decreased

12. Nonblood therapy is the treatment of choice to avoid risks associated with component transfusion (hepatitis, HIV). Desmopressin, DDAVP, a synthetic vasopressin used to treat diabetes insipidus, increases the release of both von Willebrand's factor (vWF) and VIII:C from the endothelial cells lining the blood vessels and is most effective in Type 1 vWD. Type III vWF patients do not respond (no elevation or only slightly increased vWF and

VIII:C). Type IIb patients may release abnormal vWF, which can bind with platelets causing an increased clearance, leading to thrombocytopenia.

13. Components of choice for von Willebrand's disease are some FVIII concentrates, cryoprecipitate, and vWF. Cryoprecipitate contains 1000 to 1250 U of factor VIII:C, and the dosage is usually 10 bags. Humate-P and Koate-HS are examples of brand names of FVIII concentrate.

BLOOD BANK CASE 1–9 ANSWERS

1. No, the results provide no indication of in vitro hemolysis. The pre- and post-transfusion urine and serum specimens were negative for visible hemolysis. The direct antiglobulin tests and antibody screens were also negative on both specimens. The results of both pre- and post-transfusion direct antiglobulin and antibody screens were included in this case study, although many laboratories routinely perform these tests only on the post-transfusion specimen unless the post-transfusion sample is positive on either test.

2. Pat is negative for alloantibodies (antibody screening cells are negative) and autoantibodies (negative autocontrol).

3. Pat did have a transfusion reaction. The fever and chills associated with negative antibody screen and direct antiglobulin tests point to a febrile nonhemolytic transfusion reaction (FNHTR).

4. FNHTRs are characterized by fever (temperature 1°C or more above the pretransfusion temperature within 8 to 24 hours of transfusion) and sometimes chills. Other less common symptoms are nausea, vomiting, headache, and back pain.

5. The symptoms are most often caused by human leukocyte antigens (HLAs) antibodies in the patient's serum reacting with leukocytes or platelets in the donor's blood. Cytokines released by white blood cells (WBCs) during storage may also be responsible for an FNHTR. Cytokines are proteins secreted by various cells (mostly leukocytes) that regulate the immune response's intensity and duration by changing the cells that produce them and the cells around them. FNHTR occurs in 0.5%–1.0% of RBC transfusions.

6. The following data may prove helpful in determining the type/source of the transfusion reaction:
   a. What is the patient's diagnosis?
   b. Has the patient had any previous transfusions?
   c. If the patient is female, has she ever been pregnant including live births and miscarriages? If so, how many?
   d. Is the patient on any medications?
   e. What were the signs or symptoms that led to the suspicion of a transfusion reaction?

7. a. No, FNHTRs are not life-threatening.
   b. However, the symptoms are also found in early acute hemolytic reactions or following transfusion of a bacterially contaminated blood

product; therefore, care must be taken to differentiate febrile non-hemolytic from these more serious, life-threatening reactions.

8. Pretreatment with antipyretics, e.g., acetaminophen, will sometimes prevent FNHTR. If not, the patient should be transfused with leukocyte-reduced RBCs. Reduction of WBCs to less than $5 \times 10^6/U$ will prevent most cases of FNHTR.

9. The incidence of FNHTR is increased in patients who have had multiple transfusions and women with multiple pregnancies.

10. Additional tests that may be indicated if any of the preliminary workup is positive:

    a. Possibility of a clerical error

        i. ABO grouping and Rh on pre- and post-transfusion specimens

    b. Possibility of new antibody(ies)

        i. Major compatibility tests on pre- and post-transfusion specimens

        ii. Alloantibody identification, if antibody screen is positive

        iii. Antigen typing, if alloantibody is identified

    c. Hemolytic process

        i. Hemoglobin/hematocrit

        ii. Unconjugated (indirect) bilirubin 5 to 7 hours post-transfusion

        iii. Free hemoglobin in first-voided urine post-transfusion

        iv. Haptoglobin

    d. Bacterial contamination or nonimmune hemolytic process

        i. Visual inspection of donor unit

        ii. Gram stain/blood culture

Other tests may be ordered depending on the results of these procedures.

BLOOD BANK CASE 1–10 ANSWERS

1. A direct antiglobulin test (DAT) should be performed.

2. The results of the DAT indicate a warm autoantibody. The DAT panel is positive with the polyspecific IgG and anti-IgG and negative with anti-C3 in warm autoimmune hemolytic anemia.

3. The following disorders have been associated with warm autoimmune hemolytic anemias (AIHA):

    a. Infectious diseases, e.g., viral syndromes

    b. Collagen diseases, e.g., systemic lupus erythematosus, rheumatoid arthritis, scleroderma

    c. Hypogammaglobulinemia and other immune-deficiency syndromes

    d. Gastrointestinal disease, e.g., ulcerative colitis

    e. Reticuloendothelial neoplasms, e.g., Hodgkin's disease, chronic lymphocytic leukemia

    f. Pregnancy

4. The three pieces of information are the patient's diagnosis, drug/medication used, and transfusion history. If the patient was a female, you would also want to know if she had ever been pregnant including miscarriages; if yes, how many? If the patient has received blood or blood products and/or been pregnant, there would be a possibility of an underlying alloantibody.

5. a. Absorption is the process used to remove unwanted antibodies from the serum.

 b. Warm autoabsorption is performed by incubating the patient's RBCs and serum for 30 to 60 minutes. The warm autoantibody should absorb onto the RBCs, leaving the serum free of autoantibody. The serum is then tested to ensure the autoantibody has been removed. Warm autoabsorption can be used if the patient had *not* been transfused in the last 3 months.

 c. If the patient has been transfused within 3 months, a differential/allogenic absorption must be performed. Differential absorption uses three different RBCs that match the patient's phenotype or that will absorb specific antibody(ies) from the patient's serum. The purpose of these procedures is to rule out the presence of alloantibodies, which may be masked by the presence of the warm autoantibody.

6. Yes, Paul has a warm autoantibody along with an alloantibody.

7. Paul has an alloantibody, which is anti-K (anti-Kell).

8. a. The units should be typed to find K (Kell)-negative units.

 b. Paul should be crossmatched with O-positive, K (Kell)-negative red cells.

9. No, if Paul's serum is used for crossmatching, the warm autoantibody will be present and the units will appear incompatible. To find crossmatch-compatible units, the warm autoabsorbed serum should be used to perform the crossmatching.

10. No, Paul's own cells have shortened survival because the antibody is an autoantibody, likewise, donor cells will also have shortened RBC survival. It is best not to transfuse patients with warm autoantibodies. A consultation with a hematologist is recommended. If the patient is symptomatic, as Paul is, a decision to transfuse is appropriate.

BLOOD BANK CASE 1–11 ANSWERS

Donor 1

1. a. Four results in the physical examination and medical history fall outside of acceptable limits set by the American Association of Blood Banks (AABB).

 b.

		AABB Guidelines
a. Hematocrit	12.2 g/dL	Minimum 12.5 g/dL
b. Hematocrit	37%	Minimum 38%
c. Temperature	99.9°F	99.5°F
d. Ear piercing	4 months	12 months

2.   a. Karen would be temporarily deferred for an additional 8 months because of her ear piercing (4 months + 8 months).

    b. At that time she can be reevaluated for eligibility. Her hematocrit will have to increase at least 1%, to 38%, to meet the minimum guideline. The slightly increased temperature could be as a result of the cold she is still fighting.

3. No, a cold is not a reason for temporary deferral, *unless* the donor has an elevated temperature (as in this case) or is clearly not feeling well.

Donor 2

4.   a. Mike's physical examination results are within the AABB guidelines.

    b. The only factor that might be outside acceptable limits is his "close contact with a person with jaundice or hepatitis." This would be evaluated as a possible exposure to hepatitis and temporary deferral for 12 months.

5. Medical personnel are exempt because of their work with patients, some of whom may have hepatitis. If they were not exempt, it would exclude a large group of donors from the donor pool.

6.   a. Mike is not in the exempt category (question 5); therefore, he would be temporarily deferred.

    b. Temporary deferral would be for 12 months from the time of initial contact, which in this case is an additional 9 months.

Donor 3

7.   a. One result is not within the AABB guidelines.

    b. The pulse is 105 beats/min, and the AABB guidelines are 50 to 100 beats/min. Acutane (isotretinoin) use is a cause for deferral for 1 month after the last dose.

8. The increased pulse rate may be physiologically induced by anxiety, fear, or recent physical exercise. Allow Heidi to sit for 10 minutes (trying to reassure her), and recheck her pulse for a full minute.

9.   a. Acutane would not be a cause for deferral, since her last dose of Acutane was taken 3 months ago.

    b. If her pulse falls within the range, accept, but monitor her closely for signs of anxiety. If it is still elevated, defer or refer her to the blood bank medical director.

ANSWERS FOR CHAPTER 2, CHEMISTRY CASES

CHEMISTRY CASE 2–1 ANSWERS

1. The abnormal chemistry results are elevated glucose, BUN, creatinine, potassium, cholesterol, and triglyceride. Chemistry results below the reference range are sodium, chloride, total CO_2, and HCO_3^-. Abnormal urinalysis results are glucose (3+) and ketones (3+).

2. Linda is in diabetic ketoacidosis precipitated by not taking her insulin. Her plasma glucose levels remain elevated because she does not have insulin to promote the metabolism of glucose. Fats are metabolized instead of glucose, resulting in the formation of ketone bodies.

3.   a. Diabetic ketoacidosis (metabolic acidosis) is characterized by a decrease in bicarbonate, which results in a decreased pH.

     b. The deep, rapid breathing called Kussmaul-Kien respiration is characteristic of patients in diabetic ketoacidosis. This is a compensatory mechanism to blow off carbon dioxide through hyperventilation. The body is trying to correct the bicarbonate/carbon dioxide ratio back to 20/1.

     c. Ketones (acetone) being released in the expired air are responsible for the fruity odor on her breath. The excess production of ketone bodies and metabolic acidosis is most probably the cause of her coma.

4. The glucose is elevated because there is no insulin or not enough insulin in circulation to facilitate the transport of glucose into the cells.

5. Linda is a Type 1 diabetic (insulin-dependent). Type 1 diabetics are (a) often, but not always, juvenile-onset (75% are less than 30 years of age at diagnosis, so adult onset is possible); (b) prone to ketosis; and (c) insulin dependent. Onset of symptoms in Type 1 is usually abrupt (acute). Type 2 diabetics are often adult onset, are *not* prone to ketosis, are often *not* insulin dependent, and their disease is characterized by an insidious onset of symptoms.

6. The three ketone bodies are

    a. Acetone

    b. Diacetic (acetoacetic) acid

    c. β-hydroxybutyric acid

7. β-hydroxybutyric acid is not measured by any routine urinalysis procedure.

8. In diabetic ketoacidosis, sodium and potassium are usually decreased because of polyuria and excretion of salts of the acids produced by the utilization of lipids for energy. There is also a shift of water from intracellular to extracellular because of the hyperglycemia. In this patient, the potassium is slightly increased. Even though the total body potassium may be depleted, there is probably some shifting of intracellular potassium to extracellular fluid, resulting in the apparent increase. The chloride is decreased because (a) it is passively excreted with sodium and (b) much of the patient's chloride normally found in her stomach has been lost because of the vomiting.

9. mOsm/L = 2Na + Glucose ÷ 20 + BUN ÷ 3 =
   2(129) + 430 ÷ 20 + 43 ÷ 3 = 294 mOsmol/L (275–295 mOsm/L)

   In diabetic ketoacidosis, the osmolality is often at the high end of the reference range because of the high glucose.

10. Glycohemoglobin or glycated hemoglobin would provide the physician with an estimate of her average glucose level over the past 6 to 8 weeks.

11. The elevation in BUN and creatinine could be as a result of dehydration from the vomiting. The second explanation is diabetic nephropathy, which is caused by damage to the glomerulus and capillaries associated with the glomerulus. This results in a reduction in the filtering capacity of the kidneys.

12.   a. Anion gap = $Na^+ + K^+ - (Cl^- + HCO_3^-)$ = 129 + 5.8 – (88 + 10) = 36.8 (37) mmol/L (R. R. = 8–16 mmol/L)

      b. The anion gap is elevated because of the increase in ketoacids (ketones), which are unmeasured anions.

13. Yes, high triglyceride and cholesterol levels are often associated with diabetes mellitus. The elevated triglycerides occur because insulin is required for the conversion of very low-density lipoproteins VLDLs (which include triglycerides) to low-density lipoproteins (LDLs). In diabetes, intermediate-density lipoproteins (IDLs) are not converted to LDL without insulin or with insulin resistance, thereby leading to increased triglycerides. A second reason is the elevated triglycerides are due to the uncontrolled blood glucose.

CHEMISTRY CASE 2–2 ANSWERS

1. Kathy's initial patient history suggests the following:

   a. The initial chemistry order would include a cardiac profile that includes troponin I or troponin T, CK-MB, total creatine kinase (CK), and possibly myoglobin.

   b. The current recommendation to rule out acute myocardial infarction is the cardiac profile (CK-MB, troponin, and/or myoglobin) at admission, 3 to 6 hours, 6 to 9 hours, and 12 to 24 hours (Burtis & Ashwood, 2001).

2. In Table 2–4, the following laboratory values are abnormal: increased glucose, BUN, creatinine, aspartate aminotransferase (AST), and slightly decreased chloride and anion gap. In Table 2–5, the blood gas results indicate acidosis with an increased PCO_2 and decreased PO_2. In Table 2–6, CK, CK-MB, and troponin I are elevated.

3. Laboratory results are indicative of an acute myocardial infarction (AMI). Myocardial infarction occurs as a result of reduced blood supply to some part of the myocardium due to partial or complete occlusion (blockage) of one or more of the coronary arteries. This results in ischemia and death of myocardial tissue.

4. Heart muscle contains both CK-MB and CK-MM isoenzymes.

5. CK is elevated 6 to 8 hours after an acute myocardial infarction, peaks 24 to 36 hours following infarction, and remains elevated 3 to 4 days. CK-MB rises 4 to 8 hours after infarction, peaks 12 to 24, and returns to normal within 48 to 72 hours. CK-MB levels do not remain persistently elevated and may return to normal levels 24 hours after a minor infarct.

6. CK-MB relative index = $\dfrac{\text{CK-MB (mass)}}{\text{Total CK (activity)}} \times 100\%$

For mass assays (immunoassays) values exceeding 2.5% (method dependent) are indicative of a myocardial infarction (a myocardial source of CK-MB). The relative index represents a disproportionately high concentration of CK-MB consistent with cardiac necrosis.

Day 1 (20:30) = $\dfrac{47.1}{668}$ = 7.1%

Day 2 (12:25) = $\dfrac{146.6}{3461}$ = 4.2 %

Day 2 (20:35) = $\dfrac{93.0}{3743}$ = 2.5%

Day 3 (12:15) = $\dfrac{24.8}{2117}$ = 1.2%

Day 4 (07:15) = $\dfrac{12.1}{973}$ = 1.2%

7. Cardiac troponin I rises 3 to 8 hours after infarct, peaks in 24 to 48 hours, and returns to normal in 3 to 7 days. Cardiac troponin T rises in 3 to 8 hours, peaks in 24 to 48 hours, and remains elevated 7 to 10 days (Burtis & Ashwood, 2001).

8. Studies support both cardiac troponin I (cTnI) and cardiac Troponin T (cTnT) with advantages and disadvantages of both troponins. Both are useful in predicting short-term mortality risk following an AMI. Cardiac troponin T appears to be more valuable for risk stratification. Risk stratification assesses a patient's outcome following a medical event, such as myocardial infarction. Studies indicate that cardiac troponin I is more sensitive in unstable angina patients, and Troponin T may be elevated in chronic renal failure and skeletal muscle injury.

9. AST is elevated following a myocardial infarction, but it is not specific for damage to the myocardium. Liver disease and skeletal muscle disease also cause an increase in AST.

10. Myoglobin can also be used to indicate myocardial damage, but it is nonspecific with elevations in many types of muscle damage. It is elevated at about 3 hours following chest pain, peaks at about 9 hours, and returns to normal in 30 hours. Myoglobin has a high clinical sensitivity and specificity when specimens are collected every 1 to 2 hours for the first 10 hours following infarction. At time zero, myoglobin's sensitivity is 55% compared to 23% for CK-MB. At 9 hours, the gap is 91% versus 41%. Myoglobin's clin-

ical usefulness is limited by the higher false-positive rate and the quick clearance from circulation.

Increased levels of homocysteine are also associated with coronary artery disease (CAD). A rare inborn error of metabolism causes plasma homocysteine levels to rise above 100 µmol/L (reference range: < 15 µmol/L). It has not been determined whether homocysteine damages the vascular epithelium or is only a marker of atherosclerosis. Affected individuals can lower their homocysteine levels by ingesting vitamin B_{12} and folate at higher than the recommended daily requirement. Screening is recommended only for families with unexplained premature CAD.

Carbonic anhydrase III is found in skeletal muscle and *not* in cardiac muscle. Carbonic anhydrase III assays are currently being developed. The ratio of myoglobin/carbonic anhydrase III differentiates myoglobin from myocardial infarction from myoglobin due to skeletal muscle injury.

Glycogen phosphorylase isoenzyme BB (GPBB), heart fatty acid-binding protein (H-FABP), and other enzymes are currently being investigated for their appropriateness as cardiac markers.

11. C-reactive protein (CRP) is an acute reaction protein that is rapidly gaining acceptance as a predictor of increased risk of AMI and stroke. Increased levels of ultrasensitive CRP may be a sensitive predictor of patients who are at high risk for cardiovascular problems in the future.

12. Kathy also has diabetes mellitus, as indicated by the increased serum glucose and positive glucose and acetone in the urinalysis report.

13. Diabetics are at higher risk for myocardial infarctions or strokes than the general population. Elevated triglycerides and decreased high-density lipoproteins (HDLs) contribute to the risk of AMI.

14. Leukocytosis ($12.0–15.0 \times 10^3/mm^3$) is indicative of tissue necrosis in AMI. It appears a few hours after onset of symptoms and lasts 3 to 7 days.

CHEMISTRY CASE 2–3 ANSWERS

1. The following chemistry results are elevated: amylase, lipase, and gamma-glutamyltransferase (γGT). The only abnormal hematology tests are a slightly elevated WBC and the increased erythrocyte sedimentation rate (ESR).

2. a. The markedly elevated amylase (AMS) and lipase (LPS) are indicative of acute pancreatitis. Acute pancreatitis is estimated to be the cause in 1 of 500 acute admissions to the hospital and is most prevalent in the 50 and over age group.

   b. Acute pancreatitis is an acute response to tissue necrosis caused by digestive enzymes (proteolytic and lipolytic) released from exocrine pancreatic cells. In the pancreas, digestive enzymes are stored in the inactive form as zymogen granules. Free enzymes are not normally present in the pancreas, but they are activated on entering the duodenum. In acute pancreatitis, the enzymes are activated prematurely in the pancreas, leading to autodigestion of pancreatic tissue. The activation of protrypsin to trypsin leads to a proteolytic attack on the gland's structure and vessels.

3.   a. The two main etiologies of acute pancreatitis, cholelithiasis (gallstones lead to cholecystitis that spreads to the pancreas) and alcoholism, account for 80% of cases in the United States.

b. Another 10% may be attributed to trauma to the abdomen, abdominal operation near the pancreas, penetrating peptic ulcer, viral infection (e.g., mumps), drugs (e.g., antimetabolites, sulfonamide derivatives, thiazide diuretics, oral contraceptives), types I, IV, and V hyperlipoproteinemias, and hypercalcemia. Approximately 10% of cases remain idiopathic. Twenty percent of acute pancreatitis cases progress to chronic pancreatitis.

4. AMS is the most common screening test, but with the development of automated procedures, LPS is also gaining favor. AMS rises 2 to 12 hours following onset of symptoms, peaks at 12 to 72 hours, and returns to normal in 3 to 4 days. Urine AMS is more frequently elevated, reaches higher levels, and remains elevated longer than serum AMS. LPS rises 4 to 8 hours, peaks at 24 hours, and remains elevated 8 to 14 days. LPS is more specific and remains elevated longer than AMS. "Reported sensitivities and specificities for amylase are 70% to 100% and 33% to 89% respectively. For lipase they are 63% to 100% and 34% to 100%" (Kaplan & Pesce, 1996, p. 564).

5. AMS is also elevated in the following conditions:

   a. Inflammation of the salivary glands
      i. Mumps
      ii. Parotitis
   b. Intra-abdominal diseases
      i. Peptic ulcer
      ii. Intestinal obstruction
      iii. Appendicitis
      iv. Cholecystitis
      v. Ruptured ectopic pregnancy

LPS is normal in salivary gland disorders and is also not as likely to be elevated in intra-abdominal disorders. Jane's grossly elevated amylase and lipase clearly point to acute pancreatitis, because in conditions other than acute pancreatitis, the AMS is usually less than 500 IU/L.

6. The WBC can be elevated in acute pancreatitis due to inflammation. The elevated ESR is a nonspecific indicator of acute inflammation. γGT is elevated in all types of liver disease but highest in intrahepatic or posthepatic biliary obstruction. In acute or chronic pancreatitis, enzyme activity may be 5 to 15 times the upper limit of normal if it is associated with hepatobiliary obstruction. In acute pancreatitis, the AST and alanine aminotransferase (ALT) levels are slightly to moderately elevated.

7. The amylase/creatinine clearance ratio (ACCR) compares the clearance AMS to the clearance of creatinine. The renal clearance of AMS is greater than the creatinine in acute pancreatitis. In acute pancreatitis, the ratio is increased more than 8% (reference range = 2% to 5%) because tubular reabsorption of amylase and other proteins is reduced. The ACCR is used to differentiate macroamylasemia secondary to hyperamylasemia from pancreatitis.

$$\text{ACCR\%} = \frac{\text{urine AMS (U/L)} \times \text{serum creatinine (mg/L)}}{\text{serum AMS (U/L)} \times \text{urine creatinine (mg/L)}} \times 100\%$$

8. a. Ranson's prognostic signs:
    i. Age > 55
    ii. WBC > $16.0 \times 10^3/\mu L$
    iii. Glucose > 200 mg/dL
    iv. LDH > 350 IU/L
    v. AST > 250 IU/L

    During first 48 hours:
    i. Hematocrit decreases by 10%
    ii. Calcium < 8 mg/dL
    iii. BUN rises by > 5 mg/dL
    iv. PO_2 < 60 mm Hg
    v. Base deficit > 4 mmol/L

    Mortality prediction:
    < 3 signs = 1%
    3–4 signs = 16%
    5–6 signs = 40%
    > 6 signs = 100%

    b. This patient has *none* of the prognostic signs; therefore, the mortality prediction is less than 1%. The odds are she will make a full recovery.

9. Four important local complications of acute pancreatitis are pseudocyst formation, ascites, pleural effusion, and pancreatic (or peripancreatic) abscess formation. A brief description of each follows:
    a. *Pseudocyst formation:* Collection of pancreatic juice enclosed by a wall of tissue. These may be palpable on physical examination. Over half of pseudocysts will resolve without intervention, but others may require surgery or drainage.
    b. *Ascites:* The accumulation of fluid in the peritoneal cavity. This can be caused by leakage of fluid from a pseudocyst or directly from the pancreatic duct.
    c. *Pleural effusion:* A collection of fluid in the thoracic cavity between the visceral and parietal pleura. This results from the spread of the inflammation through the lymphatic system into the pleural space.

   d. *Abscess:* Rare complication. Pus collects on or near the pancreas.

10. Treatment of symptoms is the primary therapy in acute pancreatitis. Intravenous fluid replacement, discontinuing any oral intake of food or drink, adequate pain medication, and treatment of any complications, if any (as outlined in the answer to question 9) are the primary treatments.

CHEMISTRY CASE 2–4 ANSWERS

1. Tom's abnormal chemistry results are increased total bilirubin, direct bilirubin, AST, ALT, and alkaline phosphatase (ALP) and decreased albumin. Abnormal CBC results include decreased WBC, RBC, Hb, Hct, and platelet count and increased mean corpuscular hemoglobin (MCH).

2. Liver disease is the most likely explanation for the abnormal results.

3. The following categories of liver disease are probable causes:
   a. Acute viral hepatitis (HAV, HBV, HCV, HDV, HEV)
   b. Chronic hepatitis
   c. Cirrhosis
   d. Alcoholic liver disease
   e. Primary biliary cirrhosis
   f. Hepatic tumors/cancer

4. The most likely explanation is hepatitis.

5. The serology results indicate infection with hepatitis C virus (HCV). The fatigue, flu-like symptoms, and jaundice are consistent with viral hepatitis.

6. Five main etiologic factors for HCV infection are
   a. Blood products or transfusion, 32.3%
   b. Intravenous drug abuse, 16.0%
   c. Sexual partner with HCV infection, 4.2%
   d. Body piercing or tattooing, 3.6%
   e. Professional contact with HCV-contaminated person or material (medical personnel), 3.3%
   f. Unknown, 40.6%

7. Groups at increased risk of HCV are
   a. Drug users who share needles and syringes
   b. People who undergo skin-penetrating procedures: tattooing, body piercing, nail manicuring
   c. People who received blood or blood products before 1992
   d. Health care workers (exposure)
   e. Kidney dialysis patients
   f. Hemophiliacs
   g. Military personnel
   h. Prisoners

8. a. De Ritis ratio (ALT/AST)= ALT ÷ AST = 373 ÷ 564 = 0.66.
    b. *ALT/AST >1:* In infectious hepatitis and other inflammatory conditions affecting the liver, the ALT is usually as high or higher than the AST, making the De Ritis ratio greater than 1.0.
    ALT/AST <1: In other conditions, the ratio is less than 1.0.
    The similar elevations of AST and ALT in infectious hepatitis are caused by the release of only cytoplasmic AST from the hepatocytes, which are reversibly damaged (they can recover). When the mitochondrial AST is released from necrotic hepatocytes, the AST increase is greater than ALT (as in this case) and the De Ritis ratio is less than 1.0.

9. Acute hepatitis results in acute injury to the hepatocytes, which leads to marked elevations of AST and ALT, slight elevations in ALP, and normal or slightly decreased albumin. An increased prothrombin time (PT) (not performed on this patient) and a decrease in albumin indicate a more serious disease and prognosis. Chronic infection occurs in 50% to 80% of all cases and is often asymptomatic. Chronic hepatitis C is responsible for 40% of all chronic liver disease involving nearly 40 million people in the United States. It is also accountable for 20% to 30% of all liver transplantations and more than 8000 deaths annually.

10. The physician can distinguish between acute and chronic infection based on knowledge of clinical history (time from the onset of symptoms). A previously positive anti-HCV with more than 6 months between tests is considered a change from acute to chronic infection.

CHEMISTRY CASE 2–5 ANSWERS

1. Abnormal results are elevated ALP, calcium, and phosphorous.
2. Liver, bone, intestine, and placenta are tissues rich in ALP. Regan (placental alkaline phosphatase isoenzyme) is associated with some cancers (ovarian, lung, trophoblastic, and gastrointestinal) and is a placental alkaline phosphatase.
3. Liver can be ruled out because all of the other liver function tests are normal: bilirubin, AST, ALT , γGT and albumin. Placenta can also be ruled out—wrong sex.
4. Bone ALP is elevated in a number of conditions.
    a. Physiological increase—growth
    b. Healing bone fractures (physiological)
    c. Rickets
    d. Bone malignancies
    These can be ruled out with further testing (e.g., x-rays), if the physician has reason to suspect that the increase is other than physiological.
5. The elevated ALP is probably a physiological increase due to bone production during a growth spurt in children. ALP is produced by osteoblasts and facilitates bone mineralization. In children under 10, the ALP is an average

of four times the adult range. Peak activity occurs in puberty (girls 11 to 12 years, boys 13 to 14 years), when ALP can be 50% higher than in younger children. Boys often have higher elevations than girls.

6. No, the calcium and phosphate reference ranges for children are slightly higher than adult levels.

Bishop et al. (2001)

Total Calcium	Child (2 to 12 years)	8.8–10.8 mg/dL
	Adult	8.6–10.0 mg/dL
Phosphorous	Child (2 to 12 years)	4.5–5.5 mg/dL
	Adult	2.7–4.5 mg/dL

CHEMISTRY CASE 2–6 ANSWERS

1. The following results are elevated on Melissa's chemistry profile: cholesterol, triglyceride, and CK. Her thyroid profile indicates an elevated thyroid-stimulating hormone (TSH) and a decreased free thyroxine index (FTI).
2. The thyroid profile with a high TSH and low FTI is characteristic of hypothyroidism.
3. Causes of hypothyroidism can be classified into
   a. Central hypothyroidism (hypothalamic/pituitary) (secondary/tertiary)
      i. Trauma, e.g., head injury, surgery in the area
      ii. Infections, e.g., abscess, tuberculosis
      iii. Tumors
      iv. Functional defects in TSH synthesis and release caused by mutations in genes encoding for thyrotropin-releasing hormone (TRH) receptor or drugs (glucocorticoids, dopamine, L-thyroxine withdrawal)
   b. Primary hypothyroiditis (thyroidal)
      i. Surgery involving the thyroid or irradiation of the area surrounding the thyroid
      ii. Chronic or autoimmune thyroiditis (Hashimoto's)
      iii. Infiltrative and infectious diseases, subacute thyroiditis
      iv. Thyroid dysgenesis
      v. Reversible autoimmune hypothyroidism, e.g., postpartum thyroiditis
      vi. Drug-induced: antithyroid agents, lithium
      vii. Peripheral (extrathyroidal) hypothyroidism, thyroid hormone resistance
4. a. Melissa's thyroid profile (elevated TSH and decreased FTI) is characteristic of primary hypothyroidism.
   b. In central or hypothalamic/pituitary hypothyroidism, both the TSH and FTI are decreased.

c. The TSH is used to classify central or primary hypothyroidism.

5. Melissa's hypothyroidism is most likely a reversible autoimmune hypothyroidism caused by postpartum thyroiditis. Postpartum thyroiditis is fairly common, with an incidence of 4% to 6% in population-based studies (Wiersinga & Degroot, 1999).

6. The recommended algorithm to screen for thyroid disease is TSH followed by FTI (or T_3 uptake and total T_4).

7. Thyroid hormone-binding ratio (THBR), or T_3 uptake, measures the number of available binding sites on thyroid-binding proteins, mostly thyroid-binding globulin (TBG). T_3 uptake (increased thyroid-binding proteins) is increased in

   a. Pregnancy
   b. Oral contraceptives
   c. Nonthyroidal illness (NTI): acute and chronic hepatitis, HIV, estrogen-producing tumors
   d. Genetic disorders

T_3 uptake is decreased in

   a. Advanced liver disease
   b. Renal disease, nephrotic syndrome
   c. Anabolic steroid therapy, increased androgens, and glucocorticoid
   d. Genetic defect
   e. TBG-binding drugs: salicylates, phenytoin, phenylbutazone

8. Some of the most common symptoms or signs of hypothyroidism are

   a. Weakness/fatigue
   b. Dry, pale skin
   c. Memory and mental impairment/decreased concentration
   d. Hoarseness
   e. Cold intolerance (always cold even though everyone else is comfortable)
   f. Decreased sweating
   g. Thick tongue
   h. Edema of face
   i. Coarseness/loss of hair
   j. Constipation
   k. Depression
   l. Gain in weight
   m. Menorrhagia
   n. Goiter
   o. Muscle cramps/aches
   p. Edema of the eyelids
   q. Growth retardation

9. Thyroid antibodies including antithyroid peroxidase (anti-TPO) (formerly thyroid antimicrosomal antibodies), antithyroglobulin (anti-Tg), and thyrotropin receptor (TSHR) antibodies might provide further evidence for the diagnosis. Thyroglobulin antibodies (anti-Tg) are found in 85% of patients with Hashimoto's disease and 95% of those with idiopathic myxedema, and they can be found in hypothyroidism as well as hyperthyroidism. Thryoglobulin antibodies are inconclusive and do not correlate well with thyroid disease. Antithyroid peroxidase is more sensitive and specific. TPO antibodies bind with the microsomal antigens in the follicular cells lining the microsomal membrane. They interact with lymphocytic killer cells resulting in tissue destruction. Anti-TPO is found in almost all patients with Hashimoto's thyroiditis and idiopathic myxedema and in the majority of patients with Graves' disease. Thyroid-receptor antibodies (TSHR) are classified into two categories: (a) Thyroid-stimulating immunoglobulins (TSIs), and (b) TSH-blocking antibody (TSHBAb) or thyroxine-binding inhibitory immunoglobulins (TBIIs). If the TSI is negative, the antibodies are blocking; if the TSI is positive, the antibodies are stimulating. TSI can bind so strongly to the TSH receptors that TSH is prevented from binding to the thyroid membranes (Bishop, 2001, p. 411). In other words, some cause thyroid simulation (TSI), and others have no effect or decrease the secretion of thyroid hormone by blocking the action of TSH.

10. The elevated cholesterol, triglyceride, and CK are consistent with a diagnosis of hypothyroidism. The increased cholesterol is due to an increase of LDL cholesterol, which is cleared from circulation less efficiently because of a decreased T_3-dependent gene for the hepatic LDL receptor. Metabolism is generally slowed down. Thyrotropin increases the production of hormone-sensitive lipase, which results in the production of triglycerides. Changes in muscle fibers causing myalagias, muscle weakness, and so on also result in increased CK, which will return to normal once thyroid activity is normalized.

CHEMISTRY CASE 2–7

1. Phil's abnormal chemistry results are elevated serun urea nitrogen (BUN) and creatinine.

2. Laboratory results including normal CK-MB and troponin I provide no evidence of a myocardial infarction.

3. The BUN/creatinine ratio is BUN ÷ creatinine = 53 ÷ 2.0 = 26.5 on 2/18 and 49 ÷ 1.8 = 27.2 on 2/19. A normal BUN/creatinine ratio is between 10:1 and 20:1.

4. A significantly elevated BUN with a normal or slightly elevated creatinine is characteristic of prerenal azotemia.

5.   a. Prerenal azotemia results from a decreased renal blood flow. Decreased blood flow to the kidneys leads to less BUN filtered and excreted in the urine and a higher serum BUN.

    b. Conditions associated with prerenal azotemia include congestive heart failure (CHF), shock, hemorrhage, dehydration, high-protein diet, increased protein catabolism in fever, major illness, and stress. Heart failure is fairly common (10:1000 people), and the incidence increases with age.

6. The most probable diagnosis in this case based on presenting symptoms and laboratory results is CHF.

7. Digoxin is a cardiac glycoside used in the treatment of CHF. It inhibits membrane Na^+-K^+-adenosine triphosphatase (ATPase), causing a decrease in intracellular potassium, resulting in an increased intracellular calcium. The increased calcium in cardiac muscle cells increases cardiac contractability.

8. CHF is characterized by the inability of the heart to pump blood throughout the body. CHF can be categorized into right-sided or left-sided. Right-sided, or diastolic, CHF leads to edema of the abdomen, legs, ankles, and feet. Left-sided, or systolic, CHF results in accumulation of fluid in the lungs (pulmonary edema).

9. Risk factors for congestive heart failure include
   a. Diabetes mellitus
   b. Cardiomyopathy
   c. Cardiac disease, e.g., valve disease
   d. Hyperthyroidism
   e. Kidney disease

Secondary risk factors include
   a. Smoking
   b. Obesity
   c. High cholesterol
   d. Excess alcohol consumption

CHEMISTRY CASE 2–8 ANSWERS

1. The abnormal blood gas values are decreased pH, PO_2, and SaO_2, and increased PCO_2, HCO_3^-, and COHb.

2. Brian is in acidosis with a pH lower than the reference range (7.35 to 7.45).

3. Brian is in respiratory acidosis characterized by a decreased pH, increased PCO_2, and normal HCO_3^- (if uncompensated). In nonrespiratory/metabolic acidosis, the pH and HCO_3^- are decreased, but the PCO_2 is normal (if uncompensated).

4. Brian is in partially compensated or chronic respiratory acidosis. The primary compensatory mechanism in respiratory acidosis is to increase the HCO_3^-, which has started to occur in this case. It is not fully compensated, because the pH is not back to the reference range.

5. a. The kidney provides the primary compensatory mechanisms in respiratory acidosis.
   b. The kidney's physiological response to acidosis is to

       i. Increase the excretion of acids

       ii. Retain sodium and bicarbonate

       iii. Increase production of renal ammonia

    c. The respiratory mechanism, if the lungs can respond, is initiated by the increased PCO_2, which stimulates the respiratory center to hyperventilate (increase rate and depth of respirations) to decrease the PCO_2.

    d. The respiratory mechanism is often ineffective in respiratory acidosis because the lungs are the primary problem.

6. Yes, the oxyhemoglobin dissociation curve would be shifted to the right in acidosis and hypercapnia (increased PCO_2). Hemoglobin has a decreased affinity for oxygen, causing less O_2 to bind with hemoglobin, resulting in lower saturation. The decreased affinity also causes more O_2 to be released to the tissues.

7. Base excess or deficit is the difference between the titratable acids and titratable bases in a patient's blood compared to normal blood with a pH of 7.40 and a PCO_2 of 40 mm Hg at 37°C. It can be calculated from the patient's pH, PCO_2, and hemoglobin by using an acid–base chart (Burtis & Ashwood, 1999, p. 1122). Base excess is a positive value associated with metabolic alkalosis and indicates an excess in HCO_3^- or a relative deficit in noncarbonic acid. Base deficit (a negative value) is associated with a deficit of HCO_3^- or a relative excess of noncarbonic acid and is generally found in metabolic acidosis. The base excess/deficit is usually normal in respiratory acidosis, but it can be slightly elevated in acute respiratory acidosis.

8. To correct the pH to normal levels, the ratio of $HCO_3^-/cdCO_2$ has to be 20/1; therefore, the HCO_3^- would have to be increased to 45 mEq/L.

$$\frac{HCO_3^-}{CdCO_2} = \frac{x}{0.03 \times PCO_2} = \frac{20}{1} \qquad x = 20 \times (0.03 \times 75 \text{ mm Hg}) = 45 \text{ mEq/L}$$

9. Respiratory acidosis is associated with a pathological retention of CO_2. The lungs cannot get rid of the excess CO_2 produced by the body. Some of the most common conditions associated with respiratory acidosis are

    a. Emphysema—chronic obstructive pulmonary disease (COPD)

    b. Asthma

    c. Pneumonia, severe

    d. Pulmonary edema

    e. Congestive heart failure

    f. Morphine injection

    g. Drugs, e.g., barbiturates, narcotics and alcohol

    h. Respiratory distress syndrome

    i. Sleep apnea

    j. Central nervous system: trauma, tumors, or degenerative disorders

    k. Bradycardia

10. Emphysema or COPD complicated by pneumonia is the most likely explanation for the acid–base disorder in this patient.

11. Alpha$_1$-antitrypsin is associated with early-onset emphysema.

12. The elevated temperature is most likely due to pneumonia, which increased the dyspnea and cough associated with the compromised lung capacity of COPD.

13. *COPD* is used to refer to lung diseases that are characterized by chronic airway obstruction or decreased lung capacity. It is often a mixture of three disease processes: chronic bronchitis, emphysema, and asthma.

14. Brian is in chronic and fully compensated respiratory acidosis.

CHEMISTRY CASE 2–9 ANSWERS

1. The only abnormal chemistry result is an elevated uric acid. Abnormal hematology results are elevated WBC and ESR. (Many uric acid crystals in the urine sediment are not abnormal *unless* they are seen in freshly voided urine.)

2. The elevated uric acid, WBC, and ESR are consistent with gout. Podagra—monoarticular arthritis of the first metaphalangeal joint (MTP) characterized by intense swelling, redness, and warmth—is also characteristic of gout.

3. 　a. Two main types of hyperuricemia are overproduction of uric acid and decreased excretion of uric acid.

　　b. Examples of conditions under each category are as (Pittman, 1999) follow:

Overproduction of uric acid (10% of hyperuricemias):

　i. Hemolytic anemias

　ii. Primary idiopathic hyperuricemia

　iii. Hypoxanthine-guanine-phosphoribosyl-transferase deficiency

　iv. Phosphoribosylpyrophosphate-synthetase overactivity

　v. Polycythemia vera

　vi. Rhabdomyolysis

　vii. Exercise

　viii. Alcohol

　ix. Obesity

　x. Purine-rich diet

　xi. Lymphoproliferative disease—chemotherapy

　xii. Myeloproliferative disease—chemotherapy

Decreased excretion of uric acid (90% of hyperuricemias):

　i. Primary idiopathic hyperuricemia

　ii. Renal insufficiency

　iii. Diabetes insipidus

　iv. Hypertension

   v. Starvation ketosis

   vi. Acidosis, e.g., lactic acidosis, diabetic ketoacidosis

   vii. Lead intoxication

   viii. Hyperparathyroidism

   ix. Hypothyroidism

   x. Drug ingestion, e.g., salicylates, diuretics, alcohol

   xi. Toxemia of pregnancy

4. Risk factors associated with gout are

 a. Hyperuricemia

 b. Alcohol consumption

 c. Purine-rich diet

 d. Thiazide diuretics

 e. Genetic predisposition

5. Gout is found primarily in men and is usually diagnosed between the ages of 30 to 60. Affected men outnumber women by a ratio of 9:1.

6. Gout is characterized by pain and joint edema as a result of an inflammatory response. Polymorphonuclear neutrophils ingest monosodium urate (uric acid) and lyse. As the synovial fluid becomes more saturated with uric acid, crystals form, resulting in more inflammation.

7. The joint fluids from patients with gout are inflammatory. The WBC can be >50,000/mm^3, and the definitive finding is uric acid crystals (negatively birefringent crystals that are yellow when parallel to the axis of polarization). The crystals are often found within the neutrophils during an acute attack.

8. Purine-rich foods that should be avoided by patients with gout are

 a. Organ meats (hearts, sweetbreads, kidneys, liver)

 b. Various fish (herring, mussels, smelt, sardines, salmon, haddock, scallops, trout, anchovies)

 c. Yeast

 d. Grouse, mutton, veal, bacon, turkey, partridge, goose, pheasant

9. Three renal complications associated with gout are nephrolithiasis (kidney stones) and acute and chronic gouty nephropathy. Uric acid stones occur in 10% to 25% of patients with primary gout. Acute gouty nephropathy is found in patients with massive malignant cell destruction associated with treatment of myeloproliferative or lymphoproliferative disorders. The damage occurs when high levels of uric acid lead to precipitation in the collecting ducts and ureters, blocking the urine flow. Chronic gouty nephropathy results from the long-term deposition of uric acid crystals in the kidney. The deposits cause an inflammatory reaction, resulting in proteinuria and loss of the kidney's ability to concentrate the urine.

10. Allopurinol and uricosuric drugs are two types of medications that treat the underlying problem in gout, which is a high uric acid (hyperuricemia). Allopurinol inhibits xanthine oxidase, which impairs the metabolic path-

way converting hypoxanthine to xanthine and xanthine to uric acid, thereby decreasing the uric acid produced by the body. Uricosuric drugs increase the renal excretion of uric acid produced in the body and are useful in patients who are underexcreters. Probenecid (Benemid) and sulfinpyrazone (Anturane) are two examples of uricosuric drugs.

CHEMISTRY CASE 2–10 ANSWERS

1. The only abnormal result is the elevated cholesterol.
2. Some of the more common conditions associated with hypercholesterolemia are (Burtis & Ashwood, 1999, p. 830)
    a. Obesity/diet
    b. Alcohol
    c. Drugs (steroids, thiazides, anticonvulsants, beta-blockers, certain oral contraceptives)
    d. Diabetes mellitus
    e. Hypopituitarism
    f. Hypothyroidism
    g. Pregnancy
    h. Renal disease (chronic renal failure, nephrotic syndrome)
    i. Acute/transient conditions
        i. Burns
        ii. Hepatitis
        iii. Acute trauma, e.g., surgery
        iv. Myocardial infarction
        v. Bacterial and viral infections
    j. Anorexia nervosa/starvation
    k. Systemic lupus erythematosus
    l. Storage diseases (cystine, Gaucher's, glycogen storage, Niemann-Pick, Tay-Sachs)
3. The following can be ruled out by Mike's medical history, physical examination, and current laboratory results:
    a. Diabetes mellitus: Glucose is within reference range.
    b. Pregnancy: Wrong gender!
    c. Renal disease (chronic renal failure, nephrotic syndrome): BUN and creatinine within reference range; urinalysis is normal.
    d. Acute/transient conditions:
        i. Burns: Medical history is negative.
        ii. Hepatitis: AST, bilirubin, and ALP are within reference range.
        iii. Acute trauma (surgery): Medical history is negative.
        iv. Myocardial infarction: Asymptomatic (no symptoms).
        v. Bacterial and viral infections: Asymptomatic.

e. Anorexia nervosa: Medical history and physical examination are negative.

f. Systemic lupus erythematosus: asymptomatic.

g. Hypopituitarism, hypothyroidism, and storage diseases: Asymptomatic, further questioning or testing are required.

4. The most probable cause is diet/obesity.

5. Mike's LDL cholesterol (LDL-C) can be calculated using the Friedewald formula:

$$LDLC = TC - (HDL + TG/5) = 305 - (45 + 390/5) = 183 \text{ mg/dL}$$

Where TC is total cholesterol and TG is triglyceride.

His LDLC would put him in the high-risk category.

6. a. The LDLC cannot be calculated if the triglycerides are over 400 mg/dL because the Friedewald formula is not valid at those levels. Triglycerides/5 is *not* a valid indicator of very LDLC (VLDLC) when the triglycerides are extremely elevated, because these samples may also contain chylomicrons, chylomicron remnants, and/or abnormal VLDL, which have higher triglyceride/cholesterol ratios than normal VLDL.

b. The LDLC would have to be determined directly after separation from the HDLC through immunochemical separation, chemical precipitation of HDL, or ultracentrifugation.

7. Eight risk factors associated with coronary heart disease as determined by the NCEP Adult Treatment Panel (Bishop, Duben-Engelkirk, & Fody, 2000, p. 249):

a. Age: > 45 years for men; ≥ 55 years or premature menopause for women

b. Family history of coronary heart disease (CHD)

c. Current cigarette smoking

d. Hypertension (blood pressure ≥ 140/90 mm Hg or taking antihypertensive medications)

e. LDLC concentration ≥ 160 mg/dL, with < 2 risk factors

f. LDLC concentration 130 to 159 mg/dL with ≥ 2 risk factors

g. HDL concentration < 35 mg/dL

h. Diabetes mellitus

Physical inactivity was another factor considered by the NCEP panel; although it was not included as a risk factor, they recommended it as a "target intervention" along with diet and weight reduction (Bishop et al, 2000).

8. Mike has three risk factors: age, family history, high LDL.

9. The NCEP Adult Treatment Panel (Bishop et al., 2000) recommends clinical evaluation, including family history of CHD and dietary and drug therapy. The goal is to bring the LDLC to < 130 mg/dL.

10. Drugs used to treat hyperlipoproteinemia (National Cholesterol Education Program, 1993):

   a. Nicotinic acid/niacin: The mechanism of action is not known, but it decreases triglycerides, VLDLC, and LDLC, and it increases HDL.

   b. Cholestyramine/colestipol are anion exchange resins that bind intestinal cholesterol and prevent it from being absorbed. They decrease LDLC.

   c. Clofibrate: Its action is not known, but it decreases triglycerides, VLDLC, and LDLC, and it increases HDL.

   d. Probucol: Increases catabolism of LDL and inhibits cholesterol synthesis, resulting in decreased LDL and HDL.

   e. Other drugs are gemfibrozil, fluvastatin sodium, and lovastatin.

CHEMISTRY CASE 2–11 ANSWERS

1. Abnormal chemistry results are elevated total and direct bilirubin, AST, ALP, ALT, γGT, and cholesterol. Abnormal hematology results are elevated WBC and segmented neutrophils. An elevated bilirubin is the only abnormal urinalysis result.

2. a. Conditions whose symptoms are consistent with this clinical picture and should be ruled out (Santen, 2000):

   i. Acute appendicitis

   ii. Cholelithiasis

   iii. Choledocholithiasis (gallstone(s) in the common bile duct)/cholangitis (inflammation of the bile ducts)

   iv. Hepatitis

   v. Pancreatitis

   b. Others include

   i. Abdominal aneurysm

   ii. Gastroenteritis

   iii. Pregnancy, eclampsia

   iv. Renal calculi

   v. Myocardial infarction

   vi. Bowel obstruction

3. The most likely explanation, given Marie's laboratory results—especially the grossly elevated bilirubin—is choledolithiasis/cholangitis.

4. Yes, the elevated liver function tests (LFTs), WBC, and urine bilirubin are consistent with obstructive liver disease/choledolithiasis.

5. a. The following conditions can be ruled out:

   i. Pancreatitis: Amylase is within reference range.

   ii. Gastroenteritis: Medical history.

   b. The following require additional testing:

   i. Acute appendicitis: ultrasonogram, urinalysis

   ii. Hepatitis: hepatitis panel (A, B, C)

   iii. Abdominal aneurysm: computerized tomography (CAT scan)

   iv. Pregnancy, eclampsia: pregnancy test

   v. Renal calculi: kidneys, ureters, and bladder radiograph (KUB x-ray) with contrast media

   vi. Bowel obstruction: abdominal radiograph (x-ray)

6. a. Gallstones are usually a mixture of cholesterol, bilirubin, calcium, and mucoproteins. Gallstones are categorized into two major types: cholesterol and pigmented (black or brown). In the United States, 70% to 85% of gallstones are predominantly cholesterol (Burtis & Ashwood, 1999).

  b. Bile is composed of cholesterol, bile acids, and lecithin, which form water-soluble micelles. When the bile becomes supersaturated with cholesterol, the micelles are no longer water soluble and become lithogenic or capable of stone formation. Black-pigmented stones are mostly calcium bilirubinate and are found in patients with chronic hemolytic anemias (e.g., sickle cell anemia) and cirrhosis. In these conditions, the bile becomes supersaturated with bilirubin. Brown stones are formed by alternating layers of calcium bilirubinate and cholesterol along with calcium soaps. These are more common in the Far East.

7. a. Cholecystitis is associated with the 4 Fs: female, older than forty, fertile, and fat. In other words, four risk factors (Santen, 2000):

   i. Gender: Women are more likely to have gallstones, although men are more likely to develop cholecystitis.

   ii. Age: The incidence of gallstones, cholecystitis and choledolithiasis (common bile duct stones) increases with age.

   iii. Fertility: Pregnancy increases the risk because of the high levels of estrogen during pregnancy. Estrogen promotes the secretion of cholesterol in the bile while decreasing the excretion of bile salts. Oral contraceptives or estrogen replacement therapy may increase the risk of gallstones.

   iv. Obesity: Cholecystitis is more common in obese individuals than those of normal weight.

  b. Other risk factors include

   i. Genetic: Gall bladder disease does tend to run in families and in certain ethnic groups.

   ii. Race: Fair people of northern European descent, Hispanic. Native Americans, especially Pima Indians are also at high risk (Damjanov, 1996).

   iii. Medical conditions (e.g., sickle cell anemia) that result in increased hemolysis of erythrocytes (Santen, 2000).

8. No, Marie's stool would probably be described as clay- or tan-colored. Bilirubin from the gall bladder is not secreted into the duodenum, due to the obstruction of the bile duct in obstructive liver disease. Urobilin, which is formed from the bacterial reduction of bilirubin to urobilinogen to urobilin and gives stool its normal brown color, is decreased.

9. The urine urobilinogen is decreased, but this is beyond the sensitivity of the urine reagent strips, which would be interpreted as normal. The complete absence or abnormally low levels of urobilinogen cannot be detected by routine screening methods.

CHEMISTRY CASE 2–12 ANSWERS

1. The following chemistry tests were elevated: total and direct bilirubin, AST, ALP, γGT and ALT. The albumin was decreased. The CBC indicated macrocytic erythrocytes. The prothrombin time was prolonged.

2. The abnormal liver function tests/chemistry tests indicate a liver disease/condition.

3. Cirrhosis occurs as a result of chronic liver disease. The liver structure and functions slowly become more and more abnormal as normal hepatocytes are damaged and replaced by nonfunctional scar tissue.

4. Cirrhosis has many etiologies including
   a. Chronic alcoholic cirrhosis, most common
   b. Chronic viral hepatitis (B, C, and D)
   c. Biliary cirrhosis, obstruction of the bile ducts
   d. Inherited diseases
      i. Cystic fibrosis
      ii. Wilson's disease
      iii. Alpha$_1$-antitrypsin deficiency
      iv. Hemochromatosis
      v. Galactosemia
      vi. Glycogen storage disease
   e. Exposure to environmental toxins
   f. Drugs, medications

5. Given the physical symptoms, alcohol consumption, and laboratory results, the most likely cause is chronic alcoholic cirrhosis.

6. The liver is the site of synthesis for most proteins (except gamma-globulins and hemoglobin). The production of albumin and the coagulation factors I, II, VII, and X (measured in the prothrombin time) are decreased in the cirrhotic liver; therefore, the serum albumin level is decreased and the prothrombin time is prolonged.

7. Macrocytosis in alcoholic cirrhosis can be caused by (McKenzie, 1996, pp. 195–196)
   a. Folate deficiency (inadequate intake)

b. Liver disease (increased lipid deposits in the RBC membranes)

c. Reticulocytosis (hemolysis or esophageal/gastrointestinal bleeding and reduced erythrocyte survival)

d. Macrocytosis (toxic effect of alcohol on developing erythroblasts)

e. Folate deficiency due to inadequate intake and poor diet is the most common cause.

8. a. The abdominal swelling is caused by ascites (the accumulation of fluid in the peritoneal cavity).

    b. In cirrhosis, two major contributors to ascites are portal hypertension and hypoalbuminemia. Portal hypertension is caused by obstruction of blood flow by the scar tissue, resulting in leakage of fluid from the portal capillaries. This condition is exacerbated (made worse) by the low levels of albumin, which are important in maintaining the normal colloid osmotic pressure of blood, which keeps fluid in the capillaries.

9. The complications associated with cirrhosis are

a. Ascites: see question 8.

b. Hepatic coma (encephalopathy): Can be caused by hyponatremia, hypokalemia, or gastrointestinal bleeding (varices).

c. Hemorrhage from esophageal varices: Veins in the esophagus that burst because of the increased pressure in these vessels caused by scar tissue formation.

10. Increased ammonia levels are the most sensitive indicator of impending hepatic coma.

ANSWERS FOR CHAPTER 3, HEMATOLOGY CASES

HEMATOLOGY CASE 3–1 ANSWERS

1. a. It depends on the instrument used for analysis.

   b. The nucleated RBCs reported in the morphology are counted as WBCs by some instruments. When that occurs, the WBC count is falsely elevated and must be corrected to exclude the nucleated RBCs (NRBCs).

   c. The WBC count is corrected by the following calculation:

   $$\text{WBC count} \times \frac{100 \text{ WBC}}{100 \text{ WBC} + \text{NRBC}} = \text{corrected WBC count}$$

   $$17.3 \times 10^9/\text{L} \times \frac{100 \text{ WBC}}{100 \text{ WBC} + 13} = 17.3 \times 10^9/\text{L} \times .88 = 15.3 \times 10^9/\text{L}$$

2. No abnormalities are noted when the proper pediatric reference range is used.

3. a. The stress of birth mobilizes WBCs from the marginated pool of cells lining the blood vessels. Any situation that induces stress or physical activity will move these cells out into the flowing blood stream, where they can be sampled. Thus, when healthy infants are tested to develop reference ranges, this physiologic increase in WBC numbers is reflected in the reference range.

   b. Further, most of the marginated cells are neutrophils, so the relative number of neutrophils in newborns is higher than in other children. By 1 week of age, the total WBC and the percentage of neutrophils have both dropped significantly. Infants and children have higher percentages of lymphocytes than adults do. This is presumably due to the fact that their immune systems are encountering unfamiliar environmental antigens to which they are reacting.

4. a. The baby is anemic, with a 135 g/L hemoglobin.

   b. Based solely on the mean cell volume (MCV) and mean cell hemoglobin concentration (MCHC), which are within the reference ranges, this anemia would be classified as normochromic, normocytic.

5. a. This baby's hemoglobin and hematocrit values are within the reference range for an adult but indicate anemia in a newborn.

   b. At birth, babies' RBCs still contain a substantial component of hemoglobin F (HbF). Hemoglobin F does not bind 2,3-DPG as well as HbA, and as a result, oxygen binds to HbF better than it binds to HbA. This provides an advantage to the fetus to absorb oxygen from the mother's circulation. However, this advantage is a disadvantage at the tissue level, because HbF will not readily unload its oxygen to the tissue. As a result, the fetus must have higher levels of HbF to deliver an equivalent amount of oxygen to the tissue. Therefore, the reference ranges of infants for hemoglobin and related parameters are higher than in adults.

6.   a. The morphological description includes anisocytosis, poikilocytosis, macrocytes, and spherocytes. Newborns typically have larger cells and greater variation in cell size than adults, as evidenced by a higher reference range for the MCV and RDW (red blood cell distribution width index). This patient's RDW is within the newborn reference range, but the notation of anisocytosis is still appropriate because the cells appear to vary in size when examined microscopically.

b. The presence of macrocytes, which are larger than normal cells, and spherocytes, which appear slightly smaller than normal cells, would account for the anisocytosis and the poikilocytosis. The presence of both larger and smaller cells would account for an MCV within the reference range, particularly since the newborn reference range for MCV is higher than for adults. This is consistent with an apparently greater number of large cells (2+ macrocytes) than smaller cells (1+ spherocytes). Furthermore, though spherocytes can appear much smaller in two dimensions on a blood smear, their volume is not decreased as dramatically, and so they do not lower the MCV substantially.

Polychromasia is also noted. This is the appearance of reticulocytes on a Wright's stained smear. These cells are typically larger than normal and would be expected to contribute to the anisocytosis and macrocytosis. The presence of polychromasia would be expected in response to the anemia, as are nucleated RBCs, though the latter suggest that the anemia is severe and probably of some duration. Spherocytes suggest an extravascular hemolytic process where the splenic macrophages are removing a portion of the RBC membrane as cells pass the splenic sieve. The cell membrane reseals, but with less surface area to contain nearly the same volume, the cell cannot maintain its normal shape and must become spherical.

7. The elevated reticulocyte count is consistent with hemolysis. The bilirubin results are also evidence of a hemolytic process. The elevation of total bilirubin, due mainly to indirect (unconjugated) bilirubin, points to a prehepatic jaundice where the rate of bilirubin production from cell lysis exceeds the liver's capacity to conjugate and excrete it. The unconjugated bilirubin accumulates in the plasma and ultimately is deposited in the tissues, leading to jaundice.

8.   a. The relative reticulocyte count (e.g., percentage of RBCs that are reticulocytes) must be corrected for anemia and for the presence of young reticulocytes called *shift reticulocytes*. The correction for anemia is required because the relative reticulocyte count is an indication of what proportion of the total RBC population is reticulocytes. If the total number of RBCs is lower than normal, a normal number of reticulocytes will appear as a larger percentage and thus imply a more vigorous reticulocyte response than is actually occurring. Therefore, whenever the patient is anemic, the relative reticulocyte count must be corrected for the anemia.

b. The formula to obtain the corrected reticulocyte count (CRC) uses the hematocrit as the measure of the patient's anemia and compares it to the average reference hematocrit of 45%. (If you averaged the male and female ranges of hematocrit, 45% would be about the average, so 45% is the value that is typically used.) The formula for adults is

$$\text{relative reticulocyte count (\%)} \times \frac{\text{patient's hematocrit}}{45} = \text{CRC}$$

Since this patient is a newborn, the average reference hematocrit for a newborn should be substituted in the equation, and 51 will be used. This is determined by taking the low reference value of 42%, adding the high reference value of 60%, and dividing by 2 to find the average neonatal reference hematocrit. The formula for this patient is

$$11\% \times \frac{41.5}{51} = 9.5\% \text{ CRC}$$

An additional correction of the relative reticulocyte count is required when polychromasia is present. This is because the interpretation of the relative reticulocyte count is based on an assumption that the reticulocytes counted will mature into RBCs within 1 day. Polychromasia is caused by the presence of reticulocytes that are shifted out of the marrow before they reach the usual level of reticulocyte maturity and thus will need more than 1 day in the circulation to mature. The primary assumption of the relative reticulocyte count interpretation is violated when shift reticulocytes are present. To compensate for this, an additional correction to the relative reticulocyte count can be made. Using 2 days as the average number of days required for shift reticulocytes to mature in the circulation, the reticulocyte production index (RPI) can be calculated by dividing the CRC by 2.

$$\text{RPI} = \text{CRC}/2$$
For this patient: $9.5\%/2 = 4.8\%$ RPI

The RPI should be greater than 3% to equate to a reticulocyte response sufficient to correct a moderate anemia in an adult. A higher RPI is necessary to correct more severe anemias. In this case, the RPI of 4.8% would suggest that the response will be adequate to correct the anemia; however, it must be interpreted with caution in an infant due to the presence of fetal hemoglobin. Therefore, a transfusion to correct the anemia may be considered in a newborn when an adult with an equivalent RPI would not be transfused.

9. a. The percentage of reticulocytes can be multiplied by the total RBC count to calculate an absolute reticulocyte count, but this suffers from the same sources of error inherent in the manual measurement of relative reticulocyte counts.

b. Flow cytometric analysis of reticulocytes provides an accurate absolute number of cells that is more reliable than calculation from the relative count.

10. a. Hemolytic disease of the newborn would be a first consideration.

b. Hereditary spherocytosis could present with a similar constellation of findings.

11. Hemolytic disease of the newborn caused by an ABO incompatibility between mother and infant is typically a milder anemia than that due to Rh or other blood group incompatibilities. A milder condition would be reflected in a milder anemia, as evidenced by higher hemoglobin levels, few if any spherocytes, little polychromasia, and few nucleated RBCs on the peripheral smear. The presence of large numbers of spherocytes and lower hemoglobin suggests a more dramatic hemolytic process with polychromasia and nucleated RBCs representing the body's response to the hemolysis. Incompatibilities associated with Rh and other blood groups, such as Kell, are more likely to induce a brisk hemolytic reaction with the attendant peripheral blood evidence. However, these are gross generalizations that may be violated by any individual case. The responsible antibody must be identified using reliable immunohematologic methods.

HEMATOLOGY CASE 3–2 ANSWERS

1. The WBC count is elevated, most likely due to stress and mobilization of the marginated pool of granulocytes (see Hematology Case 3–1); however, other factors affecting the RBC and platelet counts may also contribute to the elevation. (See answer to question 2.)

The RBC count is slightly below the reference range; however, all other RBC parameters are within the reference range. In a healthy individual, this isolated finding would not be significant. However, in an individual who has experienced trauma, a low RBC count cannot be ignored. It could be a sign of acute hemorrhage.

The platelet count is above the reference range. Trauma and stress can cause release of platelets from the splenic pool, thus raising the platelet count, despite the likely consumption at sites of injury. Nearly 30% of the body's platelets are in the spleen at any time.

2. a. Two factors may account for the drop in hemoglobin. First, the patient appears to be bleeding into the urinary tract, possibly having ruptured the kidney or urinary bladder in the crash. However, even without bleeding, the patient's hemoglobin and hematocrit would be expected to drop (though not as far) with the infusion of intravenous (IV) solution. Such a dramatic drop is the result of blood loss together with the restoration of normal blood volume with IV fluids.

b. Restoration of normal blood volume with IV fluids would be expected to lower the WBC and platelet counts also.

3. a. The hemoglobin and hematocrit on the specimen collected at 45 minutes are a more accurate representation of the patient's true

hemoglobin because it was collected after normal blood volume was restored.

b. The specimen collected at admission represented a falsely elevated hemoglobin and hematocrit due to shock. Although the body does redistribute fluid into the blood vessels during shock to try to maintain blood volume, the peripheral vessels are constricted, preferentially shunting blood to the brain, heart, and kidneys. Thus, blood collected from a peripheral site such as the arm is concentrated and does not truly represent the oxygen-carrying capacity in the vasculature as a whole. The difficulty that the phlebotomist and nurse experienced in trying to access peripheral veins was evidence of this vasoconstriction.

4. a. In acute hemorrhage, there is no abnormality in the production of RBCs. The individual was producing cells of normal size and shape before the trauma, so the cells present at the time of the accident are normal.

b. However, with chronic hemorrhage, such a gastrointestinal bleeding associated with colon cancer or heavy menses, the body becomes depleted of iron over time. When iron is not readily available and hemoglobin production is diminished, the body first makes smaller cells but fills them with hemoglobin. Eventually, there is not enough hemoglobin to fill even small cells, and the cells become hypochromic. Therefore, in acute hemorrhage of a previously healthy individual, the cells appear normochromic and normocytic, but with chronic hemorrhage, the cells will eventually appear hypochromic and microcytic.

5. a. The body should respond to the anemia by increasing the rate of production of new cells. Therefore, the patient's blood picture would be expected to develop polychromasia on a Wright's stained smear, which is the evidence of reticulocytosis.

b. Hypoxia is the physiologic trigger to the release of erythropoietin by the kidney and the subsequent increase in RBC production.

c. An RBC transfusion would correct the hypoxia, so erythropoietin production would not be stimulated. No reticulocytosis would occur.

6. a. Erythrocytosis is the condition when the number of RBCs exceeds the upper limit of the reference range. The hematocrit will typically be elevated too. Erythrocytosis is either absolute or relative. Absolute erythrocytosis occurs when the RBC mass increases, taking up a larger than usual proportion of the blood volume and increasing the hematocrit. Relative erythrocytosis occurs when the RBC mass stays normal or even drops but the amount of fluid in the blood vessels decreases, thus increasing the proportion of the blood occupied by the RBCs, but the total blood volume has decreased. This results in an elevated hematocrit too.

b. Primary erythrocytosis is the condition of erythrocytosis without an underlying or contributing condition. The body produces an increased number of RBCs even without an increase in erythropoietin. Secondary erythrocytosis occurs when some underlying condition causes an increase in erythropoietin, so erythrocytosis occurs secondarily to the underlying condition.

c. Polycythemia rubra vera, a primary erythrocytosis, is a chronic myeloproliferative disease in which blood cell production occurs without regard for the normal feedback mechanisms. The RBC mass increases, though erythropoietin levels are low. It is both primary and absolute. In dehydration, the plasma volume decreases. The resulting erythrocytosis is only relative since the RBC mass is not increased and it is secondary to whatever caused the dehydration. Hypoxia leads to erythrocytosis that is absolute and secondary. The condition causing the hypoxia is the primary condition and the erythrocytosis is secondary. But since hypoxia leads to an increase in erythropoietin, the RBC mass also increases; thus the erythrocytosis is absolute.

d. When erythrocytosis occurs as a response to increased erythropoietin levels, that is considered to be an appropriate response. However, as in polycythemia vera, if the erythrocytosis occurs in the absence of an increase in erythropoietin, the response is considered inappropriate.

Table A-1

	Relative (e.g., Decreased Fluid Volume)	Absolute (e.g., Increased RBC Mass)
Primary		Polycythemia vera
Secondary	Dehydration	Any cause of hypoxia, e.g., living at high altitude, cigarette smoking, chronic lung disease

HEMATOLOGY CASE 3–3 ANSWERS

1. Microcytic, normochromic anemia with slight anisocytosis (but no poikilocytosis). Mild leukocytosis with normal platelet values.

2. a. Iron deficiency, thalassemia, and anemia of chronic inflammation/disease (ACI). Sideroblastic anemias can also be microcytic.

   b. Pathogenesis:

   i. Iron deficiency anemia occurs when there is inadequate intake of iron to meet the needs, such as the increased need for iron in growing children, or when there is slow and consistent loss of iron (usually thorough hemorrhage or bleeding) that exceeds intake. Developing RBCs that are deprived of iron become smaller, first, and ultimately hypochromic because there is not enough hemoglobin to fill them.

   ii. In the anemia of chronic inflammation, cytokines produced by inflammatory processes interfere with iron kinetics. Although the body actually has adequate iron stores, the iron is sequestered in macrophages and is not available to developing erythrocytes. The anemia is most often normocytic and normochromic, but it can be microcytic and hypochromic.

   iii. Thalassemia is a genetic disease in which one or more of either the alpha- or beta-globin genes is defective or missing. The gene defects may include frame shifts, splicing errors, and so on. When the errors occur in nonstructural genes, the rate of production, and thus the amount, of normal globin chain is diminished. Errors in the structural portion of the gene will typically lead to production of nonfunctional molecules (short chains, long chains, nonsense products) that may degrade quickly, thus producing the same effect as when the rate of production of a normal chain is reduced. Regardless of the specific cause, the result is decreased availability of globin for hemoglobin synthesis, resulting in small, pale RBCs.

3. The patient is a woman in childbearing years, therefore iron deficiency should be considered in the differential diagnosis of a microcytic anemia. A history of rheumatoid arthritis should lead to consideration of ACI (also known as the anemia of chronic disease).

4. The RDW can provide a first suggestion of the diagnosis. In iron deficiency, the RDW is elevated, while it is typically within the reference range in thalassemia and ACI. The variability of the RDW in iron deficiency is likely due to the variability of iron distribution in the marrow. As the iron deficiency develops, some developing RBCs will be able to access iron (and thus be normal in size), while others are located in areas of the marrow that are devoid of iron, so they become microcytic. In thalassemia, all cells possess the same genetic defect and therefore would be expected to produce cells of relatively uniform size, though not necessarily normal. In ACI, all cells can be expected to affected roughly equally by the defect in iron kinetics.

5.   a. Iron studies may help differentiate among the microcytic anemias. Further, RBC zinc protoporphyrin and serum transferrin receptor may be helpful in situations where the diagnosis is not clear.

    b. During inflammatory disease, ferritin, one of the acute-phase proteins, can be elevated, masking iron deficiency. In such cases, measurement of serum transferrin receptors may reveal the underlying iron deficiency. The Table A–2 indicates classically expected values for iron studies and other assays mentioned previously. Bone marrow sampling with Prussian blue stain will reveal iron stores. In iron deficiency anemia, iron stores will be absent. In thalassemia and ACI, iron will be present, though in ACI, it will be confined to macrophages, not erythroblasts.

■ Table A–2 ■ CLASSIC VALUES FOR IRON STUDIES AND RELATED ASSAYS

Condition	Total Serum Iron	Total Iron-Binding Capacity	Percent Transferrin Saturation	Ferritin	Zinc Protopor-phyrin	Serum Transferrin Receptor
Iron deficiency	↓	↑	↓	↓	↑	↑
Anemia of chronic inflammation	↓	↓	↓	N	↑	N
Thalassemia	↑	N	↑	↑	N	N

Abbreviations: ↓ = decreased; ↑ = increased; N = within reference ranges

6. Total serum iron is determined by releasing the iron from transferrin using acid, then forming a colored compound by reaction with ferrozine.

   Total iron binding capacity is an indirect measure of transferrin. The serum is saturated with iron to fill all transferrin binding sites. After removing the excess iron, the iron bound to transferrin is measured using the same procedure as for total serum iron. The amount of transferrin is expressed in iron units as the iron-binding capacity.

   The degree to which the transferrin-binding sites are saturated with iron is calculated by dividing the total serum iron by the binding capacity. It is expressed as a percentage.

   Ferritin reflects the levels of stored iron and is measured in serum using an immunoassay. Zinc proptoporphyrin forms when iron cannot be incorporated into heme.

   Zinc substitutes preferrentially, and the complex can be measured fluorometrically.

   Serum transferrin receptors are shed from cells into the serum. Their levels reflect the levels on the cell surfaces. When iron is scarce, cells increase production of transferrin receptors, so levels rise in serum. The receptors can be measured by immunoassay.

7. Ferritin is an acute-phase protein that is elevated in inflammatory conditions. Since the patient has a chronic inflammatory disease, the ferritin results may not be an accurate reflection of iron stores.

8. Serum transferrin receptor: Jean's level of serum transferrin receptor was 3.1 mg/L (reference range, 1.3–3.3 mg/L), and the physician determined that iron supplementation was not indicated.

HEMATOLOGY CASE 3–4 ANSWERS

1. The activated partial thromboplastin time (APTT) uses a negatively charged activator such as kaolin to initiate clotting via a conformational change in factor XII. The activator with phospholipid is provided (e.g., partial thromboplastin), and the reaction is permitted to incubate for approximately 2 minutes before the addition of calcium chloride, which allows the clotting process to complete. The time needed for clotting to occur after the addition of calcium chloride is the APTT.

   The prothrombin time (PT) reagent is thromboplastin (e.g., tissue factor) with calcium chloride already added. The addition of plasma stimulates clotting via factor VII. The time necessary for clotting to occur is the PT.

2. a. A normal platelet count and bleeding time reduce the likelihood that decreased platelet number or function are the affected portion of the hemostatic system for Ryan. The normal PT suggests that factor VII (called the extrinsic pathway) and factors I, II, V, or X (traditionally called the common pathway) are intact. The prolongation of the APTT suggests that the problem lies with the contact factors XII, XI, IX, or VIII (traditionally called *the intrinsic pathway*) or the common pathway. However, the normal PT indicates an intact common pathway.

    b. Therefore, the problem is likely in the contact pathway: factors XII, XI, IX, and VIII.

       The designations intrinsic, extrinsic, and common pathways are somewhat outdated, as it is known that *in vivo* the hemostatic process is not so dichotomous. For example, factor VII of the extrinsic pathway has significant activity with factor IX of the intrinsic pathway. However, the APTT and PT, by virtue of the relative sensitivities of the reagents to various factors and the excesses of reagent used, produce results that support the intrinsic, extrinsic, and common pathway view of the coagulation system. Therefore, the terminology is used when referring to results of such tests and their significance. However, it is not considered appropriate terminology for describing *in vivo* hemostasis.

3. Mixing studies, beginning with a 1:1 mix of patient and normal plasma used for a PT and APTT, will help determine whether the patient has a clotting factor deficiency or an inhibitor. The normal plasma can provide all necessary clotting factors, so if the test results on the mixture are "corrected" into the reference range, a factor deficiency is present. If an inhibitor is interfering with factor function, then the test results on the mixture should remain prolonged. The test may need to be incubated for 2 hours before an inhibitor will prolong the test results, or a 4:1 mixture of patient to reagent normal plasma may be needed to clearly see any prolongation.

4. Even if no inhibitor is present, the dilution of one plasma with another may shorten the clotting time as compared to the patient clotting time but not result in complete correction of the clotting test results into the reference range. For example:

Patient APTT	46 seconds
Reagent normal plasma	36 seconds
1:1 mixture	40 seconds

    The laboratory scientist is then challenged to determine whether the shortening represents correction or not. To adjust for this, the following calculation is needed (Fritsma, 2000):

    Index of correction = (clotting time of the mixture – clotting time of reagent normal plasma/ clotting time of the patient plasma) × 100

At the extremes, if the mixture has a clotting time equal to that of the reagent normal plasma, indicating obvious correction, the index of correction would be zero. If the mixture has a clotting time equal to or greater than the patient clotting time, the value of the index of correction will be high. If the index of correction is 10 or less, the mixture is considered to be corrected, while values higher than 13 are uncorrected (Fritsma, 2000). Equivocal values of 11 or 12 require collection of a new patient sample, preferably several days later.

Ryan's index of correction = 40 s − 36 s/ 48 s × 100 = 8.3 s indicates correction.

5. Since normal plasma corrected the prolongation of the APTT, it appears that the patient does not have an inhibitor. Therefore, a deficiency or abnormal coagulation molecule for an intrinsic pathway factor is the problem.

6. a. Factor assays can be performed for any likely deficiency. They can be performed using an APTT or a PT, whichever test will be sensitive to the suspected deficiency. In this case, an APTT will be used.

    b. A factor assay is performed by mixing the patient plasma with plasma known to be deficient in the factor of interest. Since the factor-deficient plasma has a prolonged clotting time, the time will be corrected if the patient plasma possesses that factor. A reagent plasma with known factor activity is diluted and also mixed with the deficient plasma. The clotting time results on these mixtures can be used to create a standard curve of percent factor activity versus time (in seconds) on log/log or log/linear graph paper. The percentage of the factor present in the patient plasma can be determined from the graph.

7. *First:* Factor VIII. This is the most frequent hereditary factor deficiency, and it is seen in males, so it would be sensible to do this test on this patient. *Second:* Factor IX. This is the next most frequent hereditary factor deficiency, and it is seen in males, so it would be sensible to test this next. *Third:* Factor XI. This deficiency is less common than factors VIII and IX, but if the first two were both normal, this would be the next factor to test. Factor XII testing is not indicated, as the patient experienced a bleeding episode that factor XII-deficient patients do not experience

8. a. Factor IX, Christmas factor.

    b. Hemophilia B.

9. See Table A–3.

■ Table A–3 ■   COMPARISON OF HEMOPHILIAS A AND B

	Hemophilia A	Hemophilia B
a. Deficient factor	VIII	IX
b. Pattern of inheritance	X-linked recessive	X-linked recessive
c. Gender affected	Males	Males

	Hemophilia A	Hemophilia B
d. Clinical presentation	Excessive bleeding may be spontaneous, postsurgical, hemarthroses	Excessive bleeding may be spontaneous, postsurgical, hemarthroses
e. Incidence	1/10,000 males[*]	1/100,000 of the general population[†]
f. Incidence among hereditary coagulation factor deficiencies	85%[*]	10%[*]
g. Treatment	Factor VIII concentrate Cryoprecipitate	Vitamin K-dependent factor concentrate

[*]Lind, 1995.
[†]Clerc, 1995.

10. a. The reference range is roughly from 25% to 120%.

   b. Mild deficiencies are typically in the range of 5% to 15% with severe deficiencies demonstrating less than 1% of normal activity.

11. Because factor assays rely on the APTT or PT that end in formation of a clot, they are essentially tests of the activity or function of a factor. Some individuals produce adequate amounts of the factor in question, but the protein is abnormal in structure and unable to react normally. In function-based assays like the APTT and PT, these individuals will appear to have a deficiency of the factor when in fact they have a defective factor molecule.

12. The clinical presentation would be the same.

13. a. Hereditary deficiencies typically affect a single factor, while acquired deficiencies are often multiple-factor deficiencies.

   b. Examples include liver disease, vitamin K deficiency or antagonist drugs, and disseminated intravascular coagulation (DIC).

   c. Acquired deficiencies are more common.

   Case summary: This patient demonstrates a mild factor deficiency that did not become evident until his hemostatic system was challenged by surgery. His family history was not known, due to adoption. However, the relatively common occurrence of spontaneous mutations of coagulation factors means that some individuals with negative family histories will be diagnosed with what are usually considered heritable deficiencies.

HEMATOLOGY CASE 3–5 ANSWERS

1. a. There is a leukocytosis characterized by a lymphocytosis. The lymphocytes are reactive in appearance. The RBCs are normochromic and normocytic but there is a mild anemia. There is a mild thrombocytopenia.

   b. The lymphocytosis is both relative and absolute.

2. A lymphocytosis with reactive morphology is characteristic of viral infections such as infectious mononucleosis (IM), viral hepatitis, and cytomegalovirus (CMV). Viral hepatitis is most likely, considering this patient's clinical symptoms, although hepatitis can accompany both IM and CMV. The mild anemia is likely the anemia of chronic inflammation, as lupus erythematosus belongs to the group of chronic inflammatory diseases.

3. Reactive lymphocytes are responding to antigen stimulation. The morphology of reactive cells reflects the transformation from quiescent typical small lymphocytes awaiting their antigens, to cells that are actively responding to antigenic stimulation with increased protein production; in T cells, lymphokines, and in B cells, antibodies.

4.
  a. A lupus anticoagulant, more properly known as antiphospholipid antibody, prolongs phospholipid-dependent laboratory tests while possibly activating platelets in vivo. The result is a thrombotic syndrome that can be characterized by arterial or venous thrombosis, miscarriages, and other manifestations, yet demonstrates prolonged screening coagulation tests.

  b. Both the PT and APTT may be affected, depending on the sensitivity of particular reagents to the antibody.

5. A screening APTT on a 1:1 mixture of patient plasma with normal plasma will be prolonged in the presence of an inhibitor such as antiphospholipid antibody. Tests that isolate the phospholipid-dependent portions of the coagulation cascade help to identify the problem. Those reactions include the activation of factors IX and X. Russell's viper venom activates factor X to Xa. The Stypven time is performed like an APTT, but viper venom replaces thromboplastin. If the reagent is diluted (e.g., dilute Russell viper venom time), the sensitivity to antiphospholipid antibodies is enhanced. Hence, prolongation of a dilute Russell viper venom time supports the diagnosis of antiphospholipid antibody.

6. Biological false-positive VDRLs may occur in the presence of antiphospholipid antibodies.

HEMATOLOGY CASE 3–6 ANSWERS

1.
  a. There is a leukocytosis characterized by a neutrophilia with a left shift and a lymphopenia. There is a macrocytic, normochromic anemia, with target cells noted. Platelets are normal in number and appearance.

  b. The neutrophilia is both relative and absolute while the lymphopenia is solely relative. The absolute lymphocyte count is within reference range.

2. The leukocytosis is characterized by granulocytosis (or neutrophilia) with a shift to the left. This is characteristic of bacterial infections and inflammatory conditions.

Inflammation elicits a systemic response that includes the release of cytokines that recruit granulocytes to the site of infection. The result is neutrophilia. To meet the increased demand for granulocytes, young cells are released early from the storage pool of the marrow and appear in the peripheral blood as a left shift.

The WBCs also demonstrate toxic changes: toxic granulation, Döhle bodies, and vacuolization. The toxic changes are evidence of activation of the granulocytes.

The primary granules of promyelocytes become diluted as they are distributed among the daughter cells and their staining properties change so they typically are not evident in mature neutrophils. The release of younger cells during infection is reflected in the staining quality of the granules that contain increased amounts of mucopolysaccharide. They stain intensely with the basic stain and result in the appearance of toxic granulation.

Döhle bodies are aggregates of rough endoplasmic reticulum (RER). They are visible because the granules of the cytoplasm do not overlay that area, and thus the RER is visible. Presumably, this is related to protein production in activated cells.

Vacuolization demonstrates that the cells are performing their function to ingest and digest foreign matter.

3. Bacterial pneumonia.

4.   a. Geoff has a mild macrocytic anemia with anisocytosis and poikilocytosis. Alcoholism is among the causes of macrocytic anemias and hence, anisocytosis. The macrocytosis appears to develop due to aberrations in RBC membrane lipids. The result is large cells that do not hold their shape well and may appear as target cells and hence the reported poikilocytosis. The macrocytes in alcoholism are also typically round, as distinct from the macrocytes in megaloblastic anemia that are characteristically oval shaped.

   b. The actual cause of the anemia associated with alcoholism is not clear. It was once believed to be associated with deficiencies of folate and/or vitamin B_{12}. The anemia may develop without vitamin deficiencies, so the inhibitory effects of alcohol on vitamin activity are possible, but since hypersegmentation of neutrophils is not seen in alcoholism, this effect is uncertain. Direct toxic effects of alcohol on developing RBCs can be seen, but the impact is unclear. Nevertheless, although it is accepted that alcohol impairs normal RBC production, the mechanism has yet to be clearly elucidated.

5. Target cells are also seen in thalassemia and other hemoglobinopathies. These conditions are typically microcytic, rather than macrocytic as in this patient.

   Macrocytosis is characteristic of megaloblastic anemia caused by folate or vitamin B_{12} deficiency but is characterized by macro-ovalocytic RBCs. Hypersegmentation of neutrophils is an early finding associated with megaloblastic anemia and is not seen with the anemia of alcoholism.

HEMATOLOGY CASE 3–7 ANSWERS

1. The CBC demonstrates a marked leukocytosis characterized by an absolute increase in blast cells. Both neutrophils and lymphocytes show a relative decrease but absolute values that are within the reference range. There is a moderate normochromic, normocytic anemia. There is a moderate thrombocytopenia.

2. Acute leukemias.

3. The patient most likely has an acute lymphocytic leukemia. The cell line can be confirmed with the use of cytochemical stains and detection of cell surface markers by immunophenotyping using flow cytometry.

4. The French-American-British (FAB) group established a classification system for the acute lymphocytic leukemias (ALLs) based on cell morphology and cytochemical staining. The three categories are summarized in Table A–4.

■ Table A–4 ■   FAB CLASSIFICATION: ACUTE LYMPHOCYTIC LEUKEMIAS*

Feature	L1	L2	L3
Cell size	Small	Mixed large and small	Large
Amount of cytoplasm	Scanty	Variable	Moderate
Basophilia of cytoplasm	Slight to moderate	Variable	Deep
Cytoplasmic vacuoles	Variable	Variable	Prominent
Nuclear shape	Regular	Irregular with clefts and indentations	Regular
Chromatin	Homogeneous	Heterogeneous	Fine and homogeneous
Nucleoli	Not visible	One or more	One or more; prominent

*Data from Lotspeich-Steininger, et al., 1992.

More recently, the Revised European-American Classification of Lymphoid Neoplasms (REAL) has classified ALL according to immunophenotyping as either pre-B or pre-T (Aster & Kumar, 1999). Both groups stain positive for terminal deoxytransferase (TdT), a DNA polymerase expressed only in pre-B and pre-T cells, thus distinguishing the cells from myeloblasts. The cells are further subclassified as B or T lineage and stage of development based on surface markers, as shown in Table A–5.

■ Table A–5 ■   REAL CLASSIFICATION: ACUTE LYMPHOCYTIC LEUKEMIAS*

Classification	Immunophenotype	Typical Clinical Features
Pre-B-cell acute lymphocytic leukemia	TdT + Lack surface Ig CD19 + CD10 +/- CD20 +/-	Predominates in children Symptoms relate to pancytopenia

Classification	Immunophenotype	Typical Clinical Features
Pre-T-cell acute lymphocytic leukemia	Tdt + CD1 + Variable expression of pan-T cell markers including CD2, CD3, CD4, CD5, and CD8	Predominates in adolescent males Presents with mediastinal masses

*Data from Aster & Kumar, 1999.

5. Myeloblasts have a finer chromatin pattern than lymphoblasts, more numerous nucleoli, and may also have Auer rods. Fine granules may also be seen in the cytoplasm of myeloblasts.

6. Hyperdiploidy is the most common chromosomal abnormality seen in ALL. Common mutations include t(12;21); t(9;22), and t(4;11). The presence of t(9;22) (Philadelphia chromosome) is correlated with a poor prognosis.

7. Early pre-B-cell acute lymphoblastic leukemia. It is the most frequent form of ALL.

8. The mechanical displacement of normal precursor cells in the marrow by leukemic cells is at least one factor contributing to the anemia and thrombocytopenia. Disruption of the normal environment of cytokines needed for cell development probably also contributes.

HEMATOLOGY CASE 3–8 ANSWERS

1. In a bacterial infection, leukocytosis characterized by granulocytosis with a left shift would be expected. Further, toxic changes (e.g., toxic granulation, Dohle bodies, and vacuolization) would be expected. The patient has toxic granulation and Dohle bodies with a left shift with a slight leukocytosis.

2. a. The notable results include
   i. Leukocytosis including an absolute lymphocytosis of generally small, mature lymphocytes with occasional plasma cells. There is a left shift of the granulocytes with toxic changes noted.
   ii. Normochromic, normocytic anemia with rouleaux of the RBCs.
   iii. Slight thrombocytopenia.
   b. Rouleaux suggests the presence of abnormal plasma proteins such as immunoglobulins that are produced in excess in multiple myeloma, Waldenström's macroglobulinemia, and occasionally in chronic lymphocytic leukemia or lymphomas. Normochromic, normocytic anemia and thrombocytopenia may accompany any of these conditions. The presence of plasma cells points to multiple myeloma as the most likely possibility.

3. Serum and urine protein studies will be important to the differential diagnosis. Determination of the amounts of various proteins is important. The demonstration of monoclonal immunoglobulins by serum protein electrophoresis (SPE) or immunofixation electrophoresis (IFE) is also needed.

Identification of the specific class of immunoglobulin as well as the presence of free light chains will also be needed. Finally, a bone marrow biopsy will be critical. The expected results in each condition are listed in Table A–6.

4. Multiple myeloma, IgG with kappa light chains.

5. a. Multiple myeloma is a neoplastic condition with no consistent chromosomal abnormality. However, a balanced translocation affecting chromosome 14 is among the most common and results in increased expression of a tyrosine kinase receptor in the malignant cells, disrupting normal cell cycle regulation. The malignant cells appear morphologically to be plasma cells and produce immunoglobulins and cytokines. Cytokines play important roles in the clinical development of the disease, especially interleukin-6 (IL-6) and IL-1β. The former stimulates late B-cell proliferation and survival, and high levels of IL-6 correlate with a poor prognosis. IL-1β stimulates osteoclasts and accounts for the bone destruction that is a hallmark of the disease.

   b. Individuals develop sharply demarcated, or "punched out" bone lesions that weaken the bone, and hypercalcemia is a result.

   c. John's low serum calcium is an unexpected finding that would be expected to rise as his disease progresses. The accumulation of immunoglobulins in the plasma contributes to renal failure and suppression of normal humoral immunity, both of which are significant causes of death.

6. Multiple myeloma patients suffer from a deficiency of effective antibody production, despite overproduction of myeloma antibodies. Granulocytopenia is also seen, though the mechanism is unclear.

7. Multiple myeloma is a disease of older adults. Men are more commonly affected than women. There is a higher incidence among African Americans than whites.

8. Immunoglobulins can accumulate in what appear like bubbles in the cytoplasm, where they are called *Russell bodies*, or the nucleus, where they are called *Dutcher bodies*.

9. The sedimentation rate of erythrocytes is affected by the negative charges on the surface of the RBCs that normally repel each other. If the repulsion is neutralized, the cells can come nearer to each other and stack together like coins. This is the rouleaux that was noted on the CBC. These stacks of cells will sink at a more rapid rate than do single cells. Proteins, as bipolar molecules, can orient around RBCs and partially neutralize their repulsive forces, thus promoting rouleaux. Increases in certain proteins, including immunoglobulins, will significantly promote rouleaux formation and thus elevate the sedimentation rate.

HEMATOLOGY CASE 3–9 ANSWERS

1. Acute leukemias.

■ Table A–6 ■ REST RESULTS IN MALIGNANT LYMPHOPROLIFERATIVE CONDITIONS

	Serum Protein Electrophoresis	Immunofixation	Bone Marrow Biopsy	Quantitative Proteins
Multiple myeloma	Monoclonal spike in the gamma region (if IgA, then bridging to beta region)	IgG (most common), IgA Free light chains common	Infiltration of plasma cells, sometimes multi-nucleate Flame cells may be seen in IgA myeloma Russell bodies and Dutcher bodies may also be seen	Increased total protein and globulin. Increased specific Ig and light chains
Waldenström's macroglobulinemia	Monoclonal spike in the gamma region	IgM	Infiltration of lymphocytes, plasma cells, and plasmacytoid lymphocytes Russell bodies and Dutcher bodies may be seen	Increased total protein and globulin Increased IgM
Chronic lymphocytic leukemia (CLL)	Small monoclonal spike may be present in gamma region	Variable	Infiltration of small lymphocytes	Slight elevation of total protein, globulin, and particular Ig
Non-Hodgkin's lymphoma	Small monoclonal spike may be present in gamma region	Variable	May not show bone marrow involvement If present, will look like chronic lymphocytic leukemia (CLL)	Slight elevation of total protein, globulin, and particular Ig

2. The French, American, British (FAB) system for classifying the acute leukemias is based on the affected the cell line, the morphological appearance of the bone marrow including morphology of the blast cells, their proportion in the marrow, and cytochemistry results. More recently, consistent genetic aberrations and immunophenotyping have been added.

3. M3: Acute progranulocytic leukemia (aka acute promyelocytic leukemia).

4. Although acute myelogenous leukemia is seen in children under 1 year of age, it is most common in adults ages 15 to 40.

5.   a. A t(15;17) translocation is characteristic of M3 leukemia.

     b. It produces a fusion gene from a truncated retinoic acid receptor-α gene on chromosome 17 and a promyelocytic leukemia gene on chromosome 15. The fusion gene codes for an abnormal retinoic acid receptor, causing interference with cell differentiation.

6. Due to the abnormal retinoic acid receptor, blast cells in M3 leukemia fail to respond to physiological doses of retinoic acid important in cell maturation. However, pharmacologic doses of retinoic acid have been shown to promote maturation of the leukemic blast cells into mature cells that are short lived and die naturally through apoptosis. Unfortunately, the effect is limited.

7. The prolongation of both the PT and the APTT suggest a deficiency of either a single factor in the common pathway or multiple factors. Single-factor deficiencies are typically hereditary, while multiple-factor deficiencies are acquired. As the patient has no history of a bleeding problem, an acquired multiple-factor deficiency is more likely. This may be due to liver disease, drug treatments, or DIC. A thrombocytopenia is common with leukemias but may also develop with DIC. Since DIC is known to occur in M3 leukemias, tests for fibrin(ogen) degradation products, especially D-dimers, would be appropriate, and the blood smear should be examined for schistocytes.

8. The primary granules of promyelocytes contain thromboplastic compounds. When the cells fail to mature and die at this stage, their contents are released and promote intravascular coagulation. Before the discovery of the effect of retinoic acid, this was a particular concern when initiating cytotoxic treatments that destroyed a large of number of blasts in a short time period, thus precipitating DIC.

9. Plasmin can degrade both fibrin, its true target, and fibrinogen. Among the breakdown products of fibrinogen are small fragments identified as X, Y, D, and E. The same fragments form with the breakdown of fibrin, but with one difference. When fibrin monomers polymerize and cross-link to form fibrin, the portion of the molecule that will be broken down to D fragments by plasmin is the portion where the fibrin molecules join. As a result, the D fragment of one fibrin monomer is bound to the D fragment of another monomer forming dimers. The presence of D-dimers is confirmation that the substrate on which plasmin is acting is fibrin and not fibrinogen; thus, clots have

formed and are being degraded. This confirms the diagnosis of DIC and distinguishes it from conditions in which plasmin may be activated without prior clotting and thus is acting on fibrinogen (e.g., primary fibrinolysis).

10. A bleeding time can be prolonged by certain vascular diseases, poor platelet function, or decreased platelet numbers. Since this patient's platelet count was dramatically decreased, the bleeding time would be expected to be prolonged and would not offer any additional information.

HEMATOLOGY CASE 3–10 ANSWERS

1. There is a marked leukocytosis with an absolute granulocytosis and dramatic left shift including a few blasts. There is an absolute eosinophilia and a relative and absolute basophilia. There is a normochromic, normocytic anemia and thrombocytosis.

2. A leukocytosis with left shift is consistent with bacterial infection, though the presence of blasts, basophils, and eosinophils is not. Also, the lack of toxic changes suggests that the leukocytosis is not due to a bacterial infection.

3. The blood picture and patient age are consistent with chronic granulocytic leukemia (CGL) (aka chronic myelogenous leukemia). In the chronic leukemias, blasts, though present, do not predominate, and there is some maturation of the involved cell series. Further, the increase of basophils and eosinophils is seen in CGL, as is thrombocytosis, at least early in the disease. A normocytic, normochromic anemia can be seen in any leukemia. CGL is most common in adults in the age range of approximately 20 to 40 years, into which Wayne falls.

4. Leukemic hiatus.

5. A bone marrow biopsy would be appropriate. In CGL the bone marrow will be hyperplastic and the M:E ratio will be increased. The predominant cells will be granulocytic precursors with increased numbers of eosinophilic and basophilic precursors as well. Chromosome studies are indicated to demonstrate the Philadelphia chromosome. A leukocyte alkaline phosphatase (LAP) stain on peripheral blood granulocytes can be done. This enzyme is missing in CGL cells, and so a low score on the LAP is consistent with a diagnosis of CGL.

6. The Philadelphia chromosome is a balanced translocation between the long arms of chromosomes 9 and 22 that places the c-ABL gene from chromosome 9 next to BCR gene from chromosome 22. The result is a chimeric gene that codes for a 210-kd fusion protein that has tyrosine kinase activity and inappropriately stimulates cell growth and division.

7. a. CGL is one of the myeloproliferative diseases.
   b. These include some relatively benign, chronic diseases: polycythemia vera, essential thrombocythemia, and agnogenic myeloid metaplasia. However, some patients' diseases convert to acute myeloid leukemias. In all myeloproliferative disease conditions, a proliferation of one or more of the myeloid elements of the bone marrow occurs.

ANSWERS FOR CHAPTER 4, IMMUNOLOGY CASES

IMMUNOLOGY CASE 4–1 ANSWERS

1. The CBC indicates a mild normochromic/normocytic anemia (mildly decreased RBC, hemoglobin, and hematocrit) and an elevated ESR. The only abnormal chemistry test is an increased gamma-globulin in the serum protein electrophoresis. The abnormal serology results are positive rheumatoid factor (RF), C-reactive protein (CRP), and a low-titer antinuclear antibody (ANA).

2. Rheumatoid arthritis (RA) is the probable diagnosis, based on Bill's history and laboratory results (positive RF, CRP, and elevated gamma-globulin).

3. Rheumatoid factor may be present in the following conditions, resulting in a false-positive test for RA:

   a. Systemic lupus erythematosus

   b. Hypergammaglobulinemia

   c. Syphilis

   d. Some bacterial and viral infections, e.g., hepatitis and infectious mononucleosis

   e. Chronic infections, e.g., tuberculosis

   f. Bacterial endocarditis

   g. Some cancers

   h. Old age

   i. Leprosy

   j. Myocardial infarction

4. Rheumatoid factor is a 19S (Svedberg) antibody with specificity for an epitope on the F_c fragment of human and some animal immunoglobulin G (IgG). It has been found in IgM, IgG, and IgA immunoglobulin classes, with IgG and IgM the most common. No, RF is negative in 20% to 40% of RA patients; therefore, it is possible to have a seronegative RA. Patients with high titers of RF do tend to have more severe and active joint disease, greater systemic involvement, and poorer prognosis for remission.

5. Elevated erythrocyte sedimentation rate (ESR) and CRP are both indicators of inflammation, infection, and/or malignancy. CRP is an acute-phase reactant that precipitates with the C-polysaccharide of pneumococcus. CRP is very similar to immunoglobulin, but unlike immunoglobulins, it is produced by the liver hepatocytes not lymphoid tissue and plasma cells. It is produced early in the inflammatory response and increases within 4 to 6 hours after surgery, infection, or other trauma. It is elevated in many other conditions. (See the answer to question 3.)

6. Yes, low titers of ANA are found in 55% of RA patients; therefore, a low-titer ANA does not rule out RA.

7. Rheumatoid arthritis has been found in 1% to 2% of the populations that have been studied, including the United States. Although the disease can

begin at any age, it is diagnosed most often between the ages of 30 to 50. Women are two to three times more likely than men to develop RA.

8. The Council of Rheumatology established seven criteria for the diagnosis of rheumatoid arthritis (Turgeon, 1996, p. 389):

   a. Morning stiffness around the joints lasting at least 1 hour.

   b. Swelling of the soft tissue around three or more joints.

   c. Swelling of the proximal interphalangeal, metacarpophalangeal, or wrist joints.

   d. Symmetric arthritis.

   e. Subcutaneous nodules.

   f. A positive RF.

   g. Radiographic evidence of erosions in the joints of the hands, the wrists, or both.

   At least four of these must be present for 6 weeks or more to confirm the diagnosis of RA.

9. Rheumatoid arthritis is an autoimmune disease. Although the etiology of RA has not been established, genetic, metabolic, hormonal, and psychosomatic factors have been implicated. A possible genetic link is the increased incidence of RA associated with Histocompatibility Antigens (HLA) II proteins, HLA-DR1 and DR4. They are found in 70% of rheumatoid arthritis patients.

   Rheumatoid arthritis may also have an infectious etiology resulting from an unusual response to an infectious agent. It is suspected that the autoimmune process may be precipitated by a bacterial or viral infection.

   Hormonal factors may also play a role. Deficiencies or changes in certain hormones may promote the development of RA in genetically susceptible people.

   It appears that RA is caused by the interaction of many factors.

IMMUNOLOGY CASE 4–2 ANSWERS

1. Mary's CBC indicates a neutropenia (WBC, 4.2). The human immunodeficiency virus (HIV) enzyme-linked immunosorbent assay (ELISA) test is positive.

2. Mary is most likely HIV positive.

3. a. The recommended guidelines include repeating the HIV ELISA; if it is positive on repeat, the confirmatory test is the Western blot.

   b. HIV ELISA usually detects anti-p24, gp120, gp16, and gp41.

   c. No, she may be too early in the infection to produce HIV antibodies, or the antibodies are not produced due to beta-cell dysfunction, which can occur in advanced acquired immune deficiency syndrome (AIDS).

4. The Western blot test is considered positive if two of the following bands are positive:

a. p24

b. gp41

c. gp120/160

If the Western blot is indeterminate (does not meet the two-band requirement but does have some characteristics of a positive Western blot), it should be repeated in 3 to 6 months.

5.   a. She is in category B according to the criteria. These include conditions that meet at least one of the following criteria: (a) Conditions are attributable to HIV infection or are indicative of a defect in cell-mediated immunity or (b) conditions considered by physicians to have a clinical course or require management that is complicated by HIV infections

    b. Examples include (Stevens, 1996, p. 285):

      i. Bacillary angiomatosis (an infectious disease causing the proliferation of small blood vessels in the skin and visceral organs of HIV patients and other immunocompromised patients)

      ii. Candidiasis: oropharyngeal (thrush)

      iii. Candidiasis: vulvovaginal, persistent, frequent, or poorly responsive to therapy

      iv. Cervical dysplasia (moderate or severe)/cervical carcinoma in situ

      v. Constitutional symptoms, such as fever (38.5°C) or diarrhea lasting more than 1 month

      vi. Hairy leukoplasia, oral

      vii. Herpes zoster (shingles), involving at least two distinct episodes or more than one dermatome (delineated area of skin stimulated by one spinal cord segment)

      viii. Idiopathic thrombocytopenic purpura

      ix. Pelvic inflammatory disease

      x. Peripheral neuropathy

6. Category C is based on the presence of AIDS-indicator conditions (Stevens, 1996, p. 285):

    a. Candidiasis of bronchi, trachea, or lungs

    b. Candidiasis, esophageal

    c. Cervical cancer, invasive

    d. Coccidiomycosis, disseminated or extrapulmonary

    e. Cryptococcosis, extrapulmonary

    f. Cryptosporidiosis, chronic intestinal (more than 1 month's duration)

    g. Cytomegalovirus (other than liver, spleen, or nodes)

    h. Cytomegalovirus retinitis with loss of vision

    i. Encephalopathy, HIV-related

    j. Herpes simplex; chronic ulcers (more than 1 month's duration); or bronchitis, pneumonitis, or esophagitis

   k. Histoplasmosis, disseminated or extrapulmonary

   l. Isoporiasis, chronic intestinal (more than 1 month's duration)

   m. Kaposi's sarcoma

   n. Lymphoma, Burkitt's

   o. Lymphoma, immunoblastic

   p. Mycobacterium avium complex of *Mycobacterium kansassi*, disseminated or extrapulmonary

   q. Mycobacterium tuberculosis, any site

   r. Mycobacterium, other species or unidentified species, disseminated or extrapulmonary

   s. Pneumocystis carinii pneumonia

   t. Pneumonia, recurrent

   u. Progressive multifocal leukoencephalopathy

   v. Salmonella septicemia, recurrent

   w. Toxoplasmosis of brain

   x. Wasting syndrome due to HIV

7. a. Four primary risk factors are

   i. Sexual activity

   ii. Intravenous drug use

   iii. Recipients of blood products (especially 1975 to March 1985)

   iv. Hemophiliacs who receive antihemophilic products made from pooled plasma

   b. She probably was infected by using a dirty needle as a result of IV drug use.

8. No, there is *no* evidence that HIV can be spread through sweat, tears, urine, or feces.

9. CD4⁺ cell counts are used to stage the progression of HIV to AIDS. Patients in the normal range (more than 500 cells/mm) usually do not have any symptoms or complications associated with HIV or AIDS. CD4⁺ counts between 200 and 499 cells/mm are associated with the infections listed in stage B (e.g., herpes zoster, thrush). CD4⁺ cell counts below 200 cells/mm are associated with AIDS-indicator conditions as classified by the Centers for Disease Control. AIDS-indicator conditions include the opportunistic infections and cancers listed under category C (e.g., *Pneumocystis carinii* pneumonia, disseminated herpes simplex virus infection). The cardinal marker of HIV-1 infection is the progressive loss of CD4⁺ T lymphocytes. The average HIV patient loses 30 to 60 CD4⁺ cells a year.

10. Viral load assays are used to determine prognosis, decide on treatment and type of treatment needed, and the efficacy of treatment. Three different HIV-1 RNA assays are on the market: RT-PCR, branched DNA (bDNA), and nucleic acid sequence-based amplification (NASBA), but only RT-PCR is approved by the Food and Drug Administration. These assays determine the number of copies of the virus per milliliter. Viral loads are highest (10^5

to 10^7 copies/mL) during the acute stage and in advanced disease. Patients with viral loads (10^2 to 10^5 copies/mL) are usually asymptomatic. HIV-1 RNA is used to monitor the efficacy of treatment. Studies (Kuritzkes, 2000) have shown:

    a. A decrease in plasma HIV-1 RNA reduces the risk of progression of the disease.

    b. The reduction in risk for disease progression or death is independent of baseline plasma HIV-1 RNA and $CD4^+$ counts.

    c. The reduction in risk for disease progression or death is independent of an increased $CD4^+$ count following treatment.

11. A rapid plasma reagin (RPR) is ordered at the time of diagnosis and should be repeated annually because of the high rate of coinfection with HIV and *Treponema pallidum*. High-risk sexual activity is involved in the transmission of both organisms.

IMMUNOLOGY CASE 4–3 ANSWERS

1. The positive RPR indicates Barbara may have syphilis.

2. The causative agent of syphilis is *Treponema pallidum*. *T. pallidum*, which is in the family *Spirochaetaceae*, varies in length from 6 to 20 μm and in width from 0.1 to 0.2μm, with 6 to 14 coils (Stevens, 1996, p. 232).

3. Three other treponemes that are rarely seen in the United States are associated with diseases. A variant of *T. pallidum* causes bejel found in the eastern Mediterranean, the Balkans, and North Africa. *Treponema pertenue* is linked to yaws found in the Caribbean, Latin America, Central Africa, and the Far East. *Treponema carateum* is the causative agent of pinta, an infection limited to the skin found in Latin America.

4. Syphilis is categorized into four major stages: primary syphilis, secondary syphilis, latent syphilis, and tertiary syphilis. *Primary syphilis* occurs after an incubation period of approximately 3 weeks, but it can range from 9 to 90 days. This stage is characterized by chancres, which are commonly found in the genital and perianal regions but can also appear extragenitally on the lips, tongue, nipples, tonsils, and fingers. *Secondary syphilis* is the disseminated stage of syphilis, where the treponemes are circulating in large numbers throughout the body. Secondary syphilis is characterized by a skin rash, low-grade fever, pharyngitis, weight loss, arthralgia, and generalized painless lymphadenopathy. This stage may last a few days up to 8 weeks, but even without treatment, it usually resolves itself within 2 to 6 weeks. *Latency* is when the patient has no signs or symptoms of syphilis, but the serological tests, e.g., RPR, are positive. The numbers of treponemes are decreased but the patient remains infectious. *Tertiary syphilis* is a slow, progressive, inflammatory disease that can occur 2 to 40 years after the primary infection. It can progress to gummatous syphilis, neurosyphilis, or cardiovascular syphilis. Gummas are lesions that can occur in the skin, bones, mucosa, muscles, and organs of the body. They are thought to be delayed

hypersensitivity reactions and may contain a few treponemes. Central nervous system (CNS) or neurosyphilis occurs when the treponemes multiply in CNS lesions. Tabes dorsalis, a degeneration of the lower spinal cord, general paresis (paralysis), and chronic progressive dementia are examples of the symptoms of neurosyphilis (Shehan, 1997, p. 215). Neurosyphilis develops in approximately 8% of untreated cases of tertiary syphilis. Cardiac abnormalities including aortic valve insufficiency and thoracic aneurysm and rupture increase the morbidity and mortality in tertiary syphilis. About 10% of untreated patients develop cardiovascular syphilis. Barbara would be classified as having secondary syphilis.

5. RPR detects reagin antibodies, which react with a suspension of cardiolipin, cholesterol, and lecithin (cardiolipin). These antibodies are nonspecific and nontreponemal and are present in other conditions.

6. Biological false-positive RPRs are found in many other conditions including
    a. Systemic lupus erythematosus
    b. Autoimmune diseases (autoimmune arthritis)
    c. Pregnancy
    d. Pneumococcal pneumonia
    e. Some chronic infections of the elderly
    f. Certain cancers
    g. Drug addiction
    Transient false-positives may also occur in hepatitis, infectious mononucleosis, varicella, measles, and malaria.

7. The physician would confirm the diagnosis by ordering a repeat RPR. If the repeat RPR is positive, a confirmatory test should be performed.

8. Confirmatory procedures test for treponemal antibodies. Four confirmatory tests for syphilis are fluorescent treponemal antibody test (FTA-ABS), microhemagglutination assay for *T. pallidum* (MHA-TP), and ELISA tests.
    FTA-ABS uses dried Nichol's strain of *T. pallidum* grown in rabbit testes, which are smeared on to glass slides, air dried, and fixed with acetone. Heat-inactivated patient's serum is mixed with a "sorbent" of Reiter treponemes, which removes antibodies to nonpathogenic strains of treponemes. Adsorbed serum is layered on the smear and allowed to react with the antigens of Nichol's strain of *T. pallidum*, and fluorescent-isothiocyate-labeled antihuman globulin is added, which reacts with the antigen–antibody complex. A positive smear has green fluorescent treponemes when viewed under a fluorescent microscope.
    MHA-TP mixes tanned formalin-fixed sheep erythrocytes sensitized with *T. pallidum* antigens with absorbed patient serum in microtiter plates or test tubes. After incubation at room temperature, agglutination of the sensitized cells is a positive reaction.
    ELISA tests use Nichol's strain of *T. pallidum* fixed to metal beads react with antibody in the patient's serum. The tracer is horseradish peroxidase-conjugated antihuman globulin IgG and the enzyme substrate, 2, 2'-azino-di(3-ethyl-2,3 dihydro-6-benzthiazoline-sulfonate).

9. The Venereal Disease Research Laboratories (VDRL) test is the only test routinely used to detect reagin antibodies in cerebrospinal fluid. It is a very specific indicator of neurosyphilis.

10. The RPR and VDRL (nontreponemal) tests are negative in late or tertiary syphilis. Treponemal tests are used to detect patients in the late stage of syphilis infection.

11. The treatment of choice for syphilis is a special long-acting injectable form of penicillin. Oral penicillin is not effective against *T. pallidum*.

IMMUNOLOGY CASE 4–4 ANSWERS

1. Abnormal hematology results are decreased WBC, RBC, hemoglobin, hematocrit, lymphopenia (decreased lymphs) and thrombocytopenia (decreased platelets). Abnormal macroscopic urinalysis results are protein 4+, blood 1+, and the abnormal microscopic results are RBCs (7 to 10/HPF) and RBC, granular, and waxy casts. Elevated serum urea nitrogen (BUN) and creatinine are noted in the chemistry test panel. Positive ANA; increased CRP, IgG, and IgM; and decreased complement levels (C3 and C4) are the abnormal serology tests.

2.   a. Given Jane's joint pain, the following conditions should be considered (MedMD, 1999):
      i. Rheumatoid arthritis
      ii. Systemic lupus erythematosus (SLE)
      iii. Mixed connective tissue disease
      iv. Myositis
      v. Fibromyalgia
      vi. Multiple sclerosis
      vii. Scleroderma

   b. Given Jane's rash, the following conditions should be considered (MedMD, 1999):
      i. Seborrheic dermatitis
      iii. Rosacea
      iii. Dermatomysositis

3. The most probable diagnosis based on the physical symptoms and laboratory results in SLE.

4. SLE is an autoimmune disease whereby the body's immune system attacks its own antigens by producing ANAs which react with various nuclear antigens. It is caused by problems with T-cell and B-cell interaction. Suppressor T-cell function is decreased, resulting in overproduction or inappropriate production of autoantibody by overactive B-cells. B cells with the CD5 marker increase in number and activity, resulting in the increased production of autoantibody. These autoantibodies react with antigens in the patient's body, forming immune complexes that can deposit in tissue and cause inflammation (e.g., proliferative glomeru-

lonephritis or lupus nephritis) or the antibodies bind directly to the cell's surface, leading to cytotoxicity or clearance of the cell (e.g., hemolytic anemia). B cells also produce cytokine interleukin-10, which has been associated with apoptosis (disintegration, programmed death) of T cells. Abnormal helper T cells, which enhance antibody production, are increased, whereas suppressor T cells are decreased. The immunological mechanisms of SLE may include the following:

    a. Polyclonal B-cell activation leading to hyperglobulinemia

    b. Production of ANA and other autoantibodies

    c. Impaired T-cell regulation of the immune response (decreased suppressor T cells and increased helper T cells.)

    d. Failure to clear Ag–Ab complexes from circulation, leading to arthralgias, vasculitis, and so on.

5. No, SLE is still the most likely diagnosis. Rheumatoid factor is falsely positive in 30% of lupus patients.

6.   a. Eleven criteria for diagnosing SLE proposed by the American College of Rheumatology follow (WebMD, 1999):

        i. Characteristic rash across the cheek (butterfly or malar rash)

        ii. Discoid lesion rash

        iii. Photosensitivity

        iv. Oral ulcers

        v. Arthritis

        vi. Inflammation of membranes in the lungs, heart, or abdomen

        vii. Evidence of kidney disease

        viii. Evidence of severe neurologic disease

        ix. Blood disorders, including low RBC, WBC, and platelet counts

        x. Immunologic abnormalities

        xi. Positive ANA

    b. Four of the criteria must be experienced by a patient before a diagnosis of SLE can be made.

7. Jane appears to have six of the criteria: characteristic rash across the cheek (butterfly rash); photosensitivity; arthritis; evidence of kidney disease; blood disorders, including low RBC, WBC, and platelet counts; positive ANA.

8. ANAs are autoantibodies found in certain conditions including SLE. They are antibodies that react against normal antigens (proteins) found in the cell's nucleus. Five different types of ANA are anti-ds-DNA (anti-double-stranded DNA), anti-ss-DNA (anti-single-stranded DNA), anti-histone, anti-Sm (anti-extractable nuclear protein-Smith), anti-RNP (anti-ribonucleoprotein), and anti-DNP (anti-deoxyribonucleoprotein). Anti-DNP is found in 70% to 90% of patients with SLE and is thought to be the LE factor (the antibody responsible for the LE cell).

9. Anti-ds-DNA and anti-Sm are found only in SLE. Anti-Sm is thought to be diagnostic of SLE.

10. The abnormal macroscopic and microscopic urinalysis results and the elevated BUN and creatinine definitely point to renal involvement in this lupus patient. Kidney disease (lupus nephritis) is present in the majority (1/2 to 2/3) of lupus patients.

11. Yes, complement levels are usually decreased in SLE because the complement system is activated, resulting in lower levels of these proteins. Levels of C3 and C4 are decreased in lupus patients and are related to the amount of renal involvement and the progression of the disease.

12. Although the cause of SLE has *not* been proven, four factors have been implicated:

    a. *Hormonal influence/estrogen:* SLE is most common in women between puberty and menopause and appears to worsen during pregnancy and immediately postpartum. Estrogens tend to enhance antibody formation, while testosterone reduces it.

    b. *Genetics:* The incidence of SLE is higher in certain families; in other words, a family history of SLE increases the risk. If someone in the immediate family, e.g., sibling, is diagnosed with SLE, the risk is 20 times greater than someone with a negative family history (WebMD, 1999). SLE patients have been found to have an increased incidence of histocompatability antigens HLA-B8, HLA-DR2, and HLA-DR3, but none of these are diagnostic of SLE.

    c. *Environmental factors:* Ultraviolet light, bacterial and viral infections (Epstein Barr) are among the factors that have been associated with inducing or exacerbating SLE. A viral infection that disrupts the T-cell population has been implicated as a possible trigger.

    d. *Drug-induced:* Certain drugs have been linked to drug-induced lupus that is reversible. Symptoms usually disappear when the drug is discontinued. Examples of drugs that have been implicated in drug-induced SLE are phenytoin (anticonvulsant), methyldopa (antihypertensive), chlorpromazine, isoniazid, penicillin, and sulfonamides (Turgeon, 1996).

IMMUNOLOGY CASE 4–5 ANSWERS

1. The abnormal CBC results are increased WBC, decreased Segs, increased lymphocytes (40+25 atypicals), and 25 atypical lymphocytes. Her chemistry profile indicates elevated total bilirubin, aspartate aminotransferase (AST), and (ALT). The serology results reveal a positive monotest.

2. Based on Tammy's history and laboratory results, the most probable diagnosis is infectious mononucleosis (IM). She exhibited the characteristic triad of fever, pharyngitis, and lymphadenopathy lasting for 1 to 4 weeks.

3. The peak incidence of IM is in 15- to 17-year-olds. It is usually found in patients between 10 and 35 years of age, but it can occur in infants and in

older patients. IM is called the "kissing disease" because it requires contact with the saliva of a person infected with the virus. It cannot be transmitted through blood or air.

4. No, a negative monotest does not rule out IM. Not everyone with IM develops a positive monotest. It is positive in 80% to 90% of adults, but as low as 10% to 40% of children. Immunosuppressed patients may also remain heterophile negative.

5. The monotest detects the presence of heterophile antibodies. Heterophile antibodies are a group of antibodies that cross-react with antigens different from the antigen that stimulated their production.

6.   a. Heterophile antibodies are categorized in three major classes: Paul-Bunnell (non-Forrsman), Forrsman, and serum sickness. Paul-Bunnell antibodies are associated with IM. Forrsman antibodies are formed in response to certain bacteria. Serum sickness antibodies are formed following injection of antitoxins derived from horses or other animals used for passive immunization against snake venom, rabies, and so on.

   b. The Davidsohn differential test differentiates between the three classes of heterophile antibodies. Paul-Bunnell antibodies react or are absorbed by erythrocytes of various species (sheep, beef, ox, and horse) but not with guinea pig kidney. The opposite is true of Forrsman antibodies (not absorbed by beef erythrocytes and absorbed by guinea pig kidney). Serum sickness heterophile antibodies are absorbed by both beef erythrocytes and guinea pig kidney.

   c. The monotest is based on the agglutination of horse erythrocytes by IM heterophile antibodies. A number of rapid slide tests for mononucleosis are based on the same principle. A differential slide test reacts the patient's serum with guinea pig kidney on one part of the slide and beef erythrocyte on the second part. Horse RBCs are then added to both sides. Guinea pig kidney will absorb only Forrsman heterophile antibodies, and beef erythrocytes will absorb only IM heterophile antibodies. Agglutination of the horse erythrocytes after absorption with guinea pig kidney and no agglutination or weaker agglutination after absorption with beef erythrocytes are indicative of IM.

7. The Epstein-Barr virus (EBV) is the causative agent of IM. EBV is also associated with Burkitt's lymphoma (a childhood cancer of the head and neck found primarily in Africa and New Guinea) and nasopharyngeal carcinoma (found mostly in southern China).

8.   a. The physician can repeat the monotest a week later.

   b. If it is still negative, tests for more specific EBV antibodies (EBV-VCA-IgM) can be ordered to confirm the diagnosis.

9.   a. The most common EBV antigens are EBV early antigen (EA), EBV viral capsid antigen (VCA), EBV nuclear antigen (EBNA), and the corresponding antibodies anti-VCA-IgG, anti-VCA-IGM, anti-EA, and anti-EBNA.

    b. VCA antibodies are the most commonly measured. Anti-VCA-IgM is produced early in the infection and gradually disappears or becomes undetectable (2 to 4 months), but anti-VCA-IgG is produced early in the infection and usually remains detectable for life. Anti-VCA-IgM is found in 97% of patients in acute primary infection and is the most valuable antibody. Anti-EA is present in acute and recent primary infection (8 to 12 weeks) but disappears and is detectable only if the infection is reactivated. Anti-EBNA is not present in acute primary infection but is detectable in recent (within 2 to 4 months) and remote primary infections (convalescent) and upon reactivation of the EBV.

10. Cytomegalovirus (CMV), adenovirus, and *Toxoplasma gondii* can also produce "mononucleosis-like" symptoms.

11. Acute lymphoblastic leukemia and malignant lymphoma have similar hematological pictures and must be ruled out by a positive monotest or EBV testing.

12.   a. The elevated total bilirubin, AST, and ALT are associated with liver disease.

    b. This is consistent with the diagnosis of IM, which often has mild liver involvement leading to mildly elevated liver function tests.

13. The incubation period is from 4 to 7 weeks. Most patients recover in 4 to 6 weeks without any treatment, although fatigue may last over 2 months.

14. IM usually requires no treatment except for rest, analgesics, and warm salt gargles to relieve sore throat pain.

ANSWERS FOR CHAPTER 5, MICROBIOLOGY CASES

MICROBIOLOGY CASE 5–1 ANSWERS

1. This is a very good-quality specimen and is very likely to provide clinically relevant information. The direct Gram's stain can be very useful in determining the clinical usefulness of specimens, particularly sputum specimens. Many methods are used to calculate the quality of sputum specimens. In general, quality is determined by evaluating the number of neutrophils ("good") relative to the number of squamous cells ("bad"). This specimen shows many neutrophils, which are positive indicators of quality and indicate an infectious or inflammatory process. The specimen also shows rare squamous epithelial cells, which are negative indicators of quality and may indicate contamination of the specimen with oral flora. Since this specimen has many neutrophils and few squamous cells, the overall quality of the specimen is very good.

2. *Streptococcus pneumoniae* is the pathogen suspected in this pneumonia. *S. pneumoniae* often appears on Gram's stain as gram-positive lancet-shaped cocci in pairs (diplococci) or in short chains. The predominant colony type described is also typical for this organism. *S. pneumoniae* is the most common cause of community-acquired bacterial pneumonia. Those at increased risk for serious infection include infants and the elderly.

3. "Greening," or incomplete hemolysis on blood agar, is consistent with *S. pneumoniae* and is called alpha-hemolysis. Beta-hemolysis is complete clearing of the media, and the term gamma hemolysis is used to describe a lack of hemolysis on blood agar.

4. Streptococci in the viridans group are also alpha-hemolytic. These organisms are part of the normal upper respiratory flora and are often seen in expectorated sputum specimens as a result of the specimen passing through the oral cavity.

5. Bile (sodium desoxycholate) solubility and optochin disk ("P" disk, ethylhydrocupriene-HCl) tests are useful in differentiating *S. pneumoniae* from other alpha-hemolytic streptococci. Colonies of *S. pneumoniae* are soluble in sodium desoxycholate and dissolve after 30 minutes incubation at 35°C, while other alpha-hemolytic streptococci are insoluble and remain intact. *S. pneumoniae* is sensitive to optochin and will show a zone of inhibition around the disk, whereas other alpha-hemolytic streptococci show resistance in this test and grow up to the disk. Specific latex agglutination reagents are also available for the identification of *S. pneumoniae*.

6. No, the patient does not have a polymicrobial infection. These organisms are part of the normal oral (upper respiratory, oropharyngeal) flora and can easily become incorporated in the sputum as it is expectorated. Viridans streptococci, nonpathogenic *Neisseria* spp. (gram-negative cocci), and *Corynebacterium* spp. (gram-positive bacilli) are often part of the upper respiratory flora.

7. Yes, antimicrobial susceptibility testing should be performed. Routine testing of isolates of *S. pneumoniae* should at least consist of a screening test for resistance to penicillin. Penicillin-resistant strains of *S. pneumoniae* are increasing in prevalence around the country.

8. *Streptococcus pneumoniae* possess a polysaccharide capsule, which helps the organism evade phagocytosis. The capsule also contributes to the "wet-looking" mucoid nature of the colonies grown in culture. The capsule is also one of the factors that stimulates the copious quantities of purulent sputum often produced by the patients infected with the organism.

9. A vaccine is available that contains capsular polysaccharide from 23 of the most commonly encountered serotypes of *S. pneumoniae*. The vaccine will elicit the production of protective antibodies in most subjects, although the response is decreased in patients with underlying disease.

10. Blood and urine cultures are often part of a routine septic workup when a patient presents with a fever. Blood cultures were collected in this case to determine if the infection had spread from the lungs. In elderly patients with severe disease, the blood cultures may be positive with up to 30% of the cases.

MICROBIOLOGY CASE 5–2 ANSWERS

1. The organism suspected in this case is *Neisseria gonorrhoeae*. The direct Gram's stain results from male patients are extremely sensitive and specific for diagnosis of this infection. It is important to note that in contrast to direct Gram's stain results from males, direct Gram's stains from symptomatic females are significantly less sensitive and specific. In specimens from female patients, it is necessary to observe the organisms within the neutrophils, but even with this qualification, the sensitivity and specificity remain significantly lower in females. Observation of the direct Gram's stain result should be considered suggestive or presumptive, and further testing (either culture or molecular techniques) should be done for confirmation.

2. The *Neisseria* species in general are very susceptible to desiccation, and measures must be taken to guard against this. Dacron or Rayon swabs should also be used, since some cotton and calcium alginate swabs can be inhibitory to gonococci. As with all specimens, timely transport to the laboratory is very important. If a delay in transport to the laboratory is expected, as with outpatient collection sites and some clinics, specimens may be planted directly onto solid media, incubated, and then transported. Several systems for this purpose are commercially available and contain selective media and individual generator systems to produce the appropriate atmosphere for growth of the organisms.

3. For conventional culture methods, selective and nonselective media should be inoculated. Several choices are commercially available for selective media to isolate *N. gonorrhoeae* and may include one of the following: Modified Thayer-Martin (MTM), Martin-Lewis (ML), GC-Lect, and New York City (NYC) medium. All of these contain agents that will inhibit most

other organisms and allow *Neisseria meningitidis* and *N. gonorrhoeae* to grow. In all of these media, vancomycin, colistin, and trimethoprim are present to inhibit gram-positives, gram-negatives and the swarming of *Proteus* species, respectively. The selective media also contain antifungal agents to inhibit yeasts and molds; MTM contains nystatin, ML contains anisomycin, and GC-Lect and NYC agar contain amphotericin B. Selective media is usually plated using a "Z" or "N" streak with the primary swab, followed by streaking with a loop perpendicular to the initial streak. Chocolate agar should also be plated with these types of specimens. This is recommended since some rare strains of *N. gonorrhoeae* are sensitive to vancomycin. Chocolate agar should be inoculated and streaked for isolation. Inoculated plates should be incubated at 35° to 37°C in a moist environment with 3% to 7% CO_2.

4. Growth on selective media and suspicious colonies on chocolate agar should be screened with an oxidase test. A Gram's stain may also be useful. Oxidase-positive organisms should be tested further for identification and speciation. Several methods are available for further testing, which may include conventional cystine-tryptic digest agar (CTA) base carbohydrates, rapid carbohydrate utilization tests, commercial carbohydrate tests, chromogenic enzyme substrate tests, and more automated identification systems, as well. Agglutination tests and other immunologic techniques are available, as are nucleic acid probes, which can be used to identify the growth in culture. Any one of these methods would be appropriate for routine identification of *N. gonorrhoeae*; however, when the isolate is being identified from a specimen from a child, it is important to confirm the identification with at least two methods. This is very important due to the social and medical–legal issues that may result from the report of *N. gonorrhoeae* from a child.

5. Some key characteristics for the identification of *N. gonorrhoeae* include the fact that the organisms are oxidase-positive, gram-negative diplococci and are glucose positive in CTA or other carbohydrate test methods. When enzymatic testing is performed, *N. gonorrhoeae* is positive for hydroxyprolyl-aminopeptidase.

6. Nucleic acid probe systems are available that react directly with the nucleic acid of *N. gonorrhoeae* and allow its detection. These systems are designed for the identification of growth from culture. Detection systems that are approved for use on direct specimens are also available. These systems include an amplification step, either polymerase chain reaction or ligase chain reaction, followed by the use of a detection method. The detection method is often chemiluminescence. Technology is available for both *N. gonorrhoeae* and *Chlamydia trachomatis*, two common etiologic agents of sexually transmitted disease (STD).

7. An advantage to using molecular techniques in this situation is the ability to detect two common pathogens. *N. gonorrhoeae* and *C. trachomatis* are often seen in the same patient population and can even be seen in co-

infection. Technology is available that will allow detection of both of these organisms simultaneously from the same specimen.

8. Since the use of direct molecular techniques does not involve cultivation of the organism, it is not possible to perform any antimicrobial susceptibility testing. Some degree of antimicrobial resistance is now widespread among strains of *N. gonorrhoeae*, and there have been reports of increasing numbers of isolates with resistance to a variety of antimicrobial agents.

9. *Empiric* means based on experience. *Empiric* in this context refers to the use of antimicrobial therapy that has been effective on many patients in the past.

10. In the case of an uncomplicated gonococcal infection, recommended therapy would be an extended spectrum cephalosporin, like ceftriaxone. The use of a fluoroquinolone can also be effective in most cases, but an increase in resistance to these agents is emerging. The combination of both agents is often recommended, since it is quite effective against both *N. gonorrhoeae* and *C. trachomatis*.

11. Both women, and if possible all of their sexual contacts, should be treated with ceftriaxone. Screening for other STDs would also be prudent. In most states, infection with *N. gonorrhoeae* is a reportable disease, and the state health department should be notified.

MICROBIOLOGY CASE 5–3 ANSWERS

1. Remember that the quality of a specimen is determined by the relative amount of neutrophils ("good") versus squamous epithelial cells ("bad"). Because this specimen has a moderate number of squamous epithelial cells and only a few neutrophils, it is considered a poor-quality specimen and would likely not provide clinically relevant data in routine situations. Poor-quality specimens should not be processed further. Processing poor-quality specimens is costly and time-consuming and does not provide clinically relevant laboratory information. *However*, since this is a specimen from a cystic fibrosis patient, it is generally accepted that an exception will be made and the specimen will be processed further. Cystic fibrosis patients will often have surveillance cultures done on a routine basis to screen for certain pathogens, and the presence of these pathogens is always significant. Therefore, the screening for these specific pathogens outweighs the usual hesitation to process poor-quality specimens.

2. Routine sputum specimens of acceptable quality are usually plated on a 5% sheep blood-agar plate (BAP), chocolate-agar plate (CHOC), and a gram-negative selective medium (like MacConkey). The CHOC plate may be omitted in some laboratories if a streak of *Staphylococcus aureus* is added to the BAP after the plate is inoculated. Additional media added for cystic fibrosis patients may include OFPBL and/or PC agar (oxidative-fermentative base-polymyxin B-bacitracin-lactose/*Pseudomonas cepacia*) and CNA agar (Columbia colistin-nalidixic acid agar).

3. As with the processing of any specimen in microbiology, media are used that facilitate recovery and isolation of the most commonly expected pathogens for that site. In the case of sputum specimens, some common pathogens that cause pneumonia can include *Streptococcus pneumoniae*, *Hemophilus influenzae*, *Staphylococcus aureus*, *Enterobacteriaceae*, and other gram-negative bacilli. There is an inherent difficulty associated with sputum specimens, since most specimens pass through the oral cavity during the process of collection and in doing so often become contaminated with normal upper respiratory flora. Recognizing the difference between normal upper respiratory flora and potential pathogens can be quite difficult for the beginning microbiologist. Media are selected that will help sort this out. Alpha-hemolytic colonies on BAP may be *S. pneumoniae*, while beta-hemolytic colonies may be *S. aureus*. Characteristic growth on CHOC and/or satelliting around the *S. aureus* streak on BAP may be growth of *Hemophilus* species. Any growth on the gram-negative selective media is usually considered significant, since gram-negative bacilli are not usually part of the normal upper respiratory flora. Special OFPBL/PC media may be used routinely to screen cystic fibrosis patients for *Burkholderia cepacia*, since colonization and subsequent infection with this organism can have grave consequences in these patients. Columbia colistin-nalidixic acid agar is a gram-positive selective media that is often used in patients with cystic fibrosis, since colonization or infection with very mucoid *Pseudomonas* or *Burkholderia* species may obscure a co-colonization or co-infection with *S. aureus*. The CNA agar inhibits the gram-negative organisms and allows the gram-positive organism to be isolated and screened more easily in these patients.

4. The atmosphere of incubation of plates inoculated with a specimen from a particular body site is chosen to encourage the growth of the most common pathogens. It is important to remember that some more fastidious organisms require a special atmosphere of incubation in order to grow. In the case of a sputum specimen, some of the common pathogens, *Hemophilus* spp. and some *Streptococcus pneumoniae*, require increased CO_2, and therefore sputum plates should be incubated at 35° to 37°C in increased CO_2.

5. As mentioned previously, a degree of difficulty is encountered when trying to recognize potential pathogens among the upper respiratory flora. It is also helpful to correlate the Gram's stain results with the culture results. For the BAP, it is helpful to observe hemolysis and screen any alpha-hemolytic colonies as suspicious for *Streptococcus pneumoniae*, while beta-hemolytic colonies are suspicious for *S. aureus*. Experience with characteristic colony morphology will also be helpful here. Latex particle agglutination testing or bile-solubility testing with sodium desoxycholate can be used to screen alpha-hemolytic colonies and identify *S. pneumoniae*. Latex particle agglutination testing or coagulase testing can be used to screen beta-hemolytic colonies and identify *S. aureus*. Characteristic "mousy" odor, colony morphology on CHOC, and/or satelliting around an *S. aureus* streak are helpful in looking for *Hemophilus* spp. Refer to the description of the colony

morphologies of the organisms that grew from this specimen; most of the organisms are part of the upper respiratory flora. Remember that this specimen was of poor quality and was heavily contaminated with respiratory flora. The small pinpoint alpha-hemolytic colonies should be screened to rule out *S. pneumoniae*, but the colony characteristics are not consistent with this organism. These colony characteristics are more consistent with nonpathogenic *Streptococcus* spp. in the viridans group. The small gray gamma-hemolytic colonies may also be nonpathogenic *Streptococcus* spp. The medium-sized, smooth, cream- to white-colored colonies may be nonpathogenic *Staphylococcus* spp. The small, clear/translucent, wet-looking colonies may be nonpathogenic *Neisseria* spp. The small, rough, "crunchy" white colonies may be nonpathogenic *Corynebacterium* spp. The large gray mucoid colonies are probably the gram-negative bacillus that is growing on the selective medium, so perhaps a quick oxidase and indole test from the BAP would be sufficient, and a complete workup would come from the selective medium. The only colonies of concern from this culture are the alpha-hemolytic colonies, and the large mucoid colonies; all of these other organisms are part of the patient's upper respiratory flora.

6. Workup from selective media, like MacConkey, should include observation of the lactose reaction. It is also sometimes helpful to perform an oxidase test on lactose-negative organisms to differentiate between *Enterobacteriaceae* (oxidase negative) and pseudomonads (mostly oxidase positive). Further biochemical tests would be required for complete identification of these gram-negative organisms. A number of commercially available manual and automated gram-negative identification systems could be used for complete identification of these organisms (API, Enterotube, BBL Crystal, Vitek, Mircoscan, etc.). Although more time-consuming and labor intensive, a battery of conventional biochemical tests can also be used to identify these organisms.

OFPBL and PC agars contain specific selective agents to inhibit the growth of most organisms (including *Pseudomonas aeruginosa*) and select for the growth of *Burkholderia cepacia* and *B. pseudomallei*. Colonies of *B. cepacia* should appear yellow on OFPBL agar due to the ability to oxidize lactose. Any growth on either of these specialized media should be identified completely using conventional or commercially available biochemical identification systems. In this cystic fibrosis patient, the presence of yellow colonies on the OFPBL agar, potential *B. cepacia*, is a reason for concern even though she has not had any serious complaints or symptoms to date.

MICROBIOLOGY CASE 5–4 ANSWERS

1. Given the diarrheal symptoms and the history of camping, parasitic disease would certainly be in the differential diagnosis. Even though the patients denied drinking water from the lake, it is possible that they could have swallowed water while swimming in the lake. It is also possible that the supply of potable water for the facility at the campground was contaminated.

2. Given the possibility of a waterborne disease, the physician probably highly suspected *Giardia lamblia*, which is the most frequently recognized pathogen of waterborne disease in the United States. Other possibilities high on the list might include *Cryptosporidium* and *Entamoeba histolytica*.

3. A routine stool culture for enteric pathogens should include a minimum of three plates. Two types of gram-negative selective and differential media should be used. One of these should allow for the detection of the lactose reaction such as MacConkey (MAC) or eosin-methylene blue agar (EMB), and one should allow for the detection of H_2S production such as Hektoen enteric agar (HE), or xylose lysine desoxycholate (XLD). These media also provide other useful information that can help the microbiologist differentiate normal flora organisms from suspected pathogens, but the two major characteristics of interest are the lactose reaction and the H_2S reaction. These plates should be incubated at 35° to 37°C in ambient air. The third plate that should be used on routine stool culture for enteric pathogens is a *Campylobacter* blood-agar (CAMPY) plate, and it should be incubated in microaerophilic conditions at 45°C. Some laboratories may also use specialized *Salmonella–Shigella* (SS) agar plates, but the use of this plate is optional and varies among laboratories. Another optional step in the stool culture workup is the use of an enrichment broth like gram-negative (GN) or selenite broth. The broth would be inoculated with the stool specimen and incubated at 35° to 37°C for 8 to 12 hours. The broth is then used to inoculate a MAC or HE and an XLD or EMB. The concept of the broth is that it will inhibit the normal flora organisms and allow the pathogens to have a growth advantage and be enriched. The use of broth enrichment is no longer recommended as routine but may be used in some laboratories or in some settings. Another optional part of processing a stool specimen is the direct Gram's stain. Physicians may request a Gram's stain to determine the presence of WBCs in the stool, an overabundance of yeast or staphylococcus, or the absence of normal flora. A Gram's stain of stool is not recommended as part of the routine workup but should be available if a physician requests the test.

4. A routine stool culture should minimally screen for the presence of *Salmonella* spp., *Shigella* spp., and *Campylobacter* spp. When reading these cultures the microbiologist observes the plates closely, looking for any suspicious colonies, which includes any lactose-negative colonies (colorless on MAC or EMB) or any H_2S-positive colonies (black on XLD or HE). These suspicious colonies may then be screened further and then identified if warranted, or identified directly, depending on the standard operating procedure of the laboratory. Any growth on the CAMPY agar is considered suspicious and may be screened further with Gram's stain and oxidase test and identified as determined by the standard procedure for the laboratory.

5. If a bloody stool specimen is received, the specimen should also be processed for *Escherichia coli* O157:H7. This testing may be considered a "reflex" test in some laboratories (a reflex test is added automatically to the

testing protocol based on significant laboratory findings), while in others a phone call may be made to the physician to recommend this testing, especially if the specimen is from a person at the extremes of age. Physicians may also request testing for *E. coli* O157:H7 when the pathogen is suspected even in the absence of frank blood in the specimen. *E. coli* O157:H7 has been seen as a causative agent of diarrheal disease in many outbreaks and in isolated cases across the United States. In some cases the infection can lead to very serious sequelae including hemolytic uremic syndrome (HUS) and death. To screen for this pathogen, the specimen is plated on MacConkey agar with sorbitol (SMAC) and incubated at 35° to 37°C in ambient air. *E. coli* O157:H7 is sorbitol negative and appears as clear/colorless colonies on this medium. Clear or colorless colonies on SMAC should be identified further. If the organism is identified as *E. coli* it should then be typed in latex agglutination tests using specific reagents developed for the somatic (O) and flagellar (H) antigens in question.

6. Other bacterial pathogens may also cause diarrheal disease, and although these may not be a part of the routine setup, testing is available when requested by the physician. When requested, the laboratory may also look for *Vibrio* spp., *Yersina enterocolitica*, *Plesiomonas* spp. and *Aeromonas* spp. in stool specimens. It is important to point out that what might be considered a special request in one region may be part of the routine in another. This is particularly true for *Vibrio* spp. and *Y. enterocolitica*. The high prevalence of these organisms in some areas has warranted that they become part of the routine setup. Thiosulfate citrate bile salts sucrose (TCBS) agar is a selective and differential medium used for the isolation of *Vibrio* spp. TCBS agar should be incubated at 35°C in ambient air for up to 48 hours. Any growth on TCBS should be screened further and identified, when appropriate, following the procedures of the laboratory. Cefsulodin irgasan novobiocin (CIN) agar is a selective and differential medium used for the isolation of *Y. enterocolitica*. CIN agar should be incubated at room temperature in ambient air for up to 48 hours. Growth on CIN agar should be screened further and identified, when appropriate, following the procedures of the laboratory. *Plesiomonas* spp. and *Aeromonas* spp. can be isolated on routine media used for stool culture. However, these pathogens resemble normal flora on these media, and the laboratory scientist must be alerted to search for these pathogens and perform additional screening.

7. A *Campylobacter* sp. is most likely the cause of the disease in these patients. *Campylobacter jejuni* is the most common bacterial cause of food-borne diarrheal disease in the United States. These organisms may be ingested in many different situations but can often be linked to raw or undercooked poultry.

MICROBIOLOGY CASE 5–5 ANSWERS

1. Infection in the third trimester, premature labor, infection of the fetus, the Gram's stain, colony characteristics and hemolysis, characteristic motility,

ability to grow at 4°C, and the esculin hydrolysis all lead toward *Listeria monocytogenes* as the etiologic agent in this case.

2. *Listeria monocytogenes* and *Streptococcus agalactiae* can be confused, in that sometimes the gram-positive bacilli can be quite short and coccobacillary (they may even chain), making them look like streptococci. The two organisms may be confused further, in that both give a positive reaction in a CAMP test with *Staphylococcus aureus*. Although *S. agalactiae* produces the classic arrow head of enhanced hemolysis and *L. monocytogenes* produces a more square zone of enhanced hemolysis, when performed under less than optimal conditions or when observed by an inexperienced clinical laboratory scientist, this differentiation may be overlooked. Both organisms have the ability to hydrolyze sodium hippurate, and the very narrow zone of beta-hemolysis around colonies on BAP is also characteristic of both organisms. It is also important to note that both organisms can be clinically significant when recovered from pregnant women and neonates. These two organisms can be distinguished quite rapidly with the catalase test, as *S. agalactiae* is negative and *L. monocytogenes* is positive. *S. agalactiae* is nonmotile while *L. monocytogenes* is motile at 22°C with a characteristic umbrella-like motility in semisolid motility medium and a characteristic tumbling motility when viewed microscopically in a wet prep. In addition, *S. agalactiae* does not hydrolyze esculin, while *L. monocytogenes* is rapidly positive for this test.

3. *Listeria monocytogenes* is quite ubiquitous in nature and has been found to contaminate many food products during preparation. Most human exposure to *L. monocytogenes* is through contaminated food. Many foods have been implicated and include raw dairy products (milk, soft cheeses, and ice cream), raw fruits and vegetables (especially cabbage and cole slaw), undercooked poultry, hot dogs and other ground meat products, and some fish and shellfish. Because the organism is rather widespread, and also because the incubation period can range from 3 to 90 days, in many cases of listeriosis, the exact source of the infection remains unknown.

4. Refrigeration is relied upon heavily as a means of preserving food and inhibiting bacterial growth. Since *L. monocytogenes* can grow at 4°C, it is able to evade this method of preservation, and refrigeration alone does not protect the consumer if the food has been contaminated in preparation. The growth of most other bacteria is inhibited quite well at refrigeration temperature. Cold-enhancement techniques have been used in some settings to increase the sensitivity of isolating *L. monocytogenes* from mixed specimens. This technique is time-consuming and is not performed routinely in the clinical laboratory setting.

5. The Centers for Disease Control provided recommendations for preventing food-borne listeriosis in 1992, and these include the thorough cooking of raw food from all animal sources and the thorough washing of raw vegetables and fruits before eating. It is also recommended that uncooked meats be kept separate from vegetables, cooked foods, and ready-to-eat-foods,

and that hands, utensils, and cutting boards be washed thoroughly after contact with uncooked foods. People at high risk (see answer 6) should also avoid soft cheeses like feta, Brie, Camembert, and bleu. There is no increased risk with hard cheeses, cream cheese, cottage cheese, or yogurt. It is also recommended that people at high risk heat leftovers or ready-to-eat foods (like hot dogs) until steaming before they are eaten. The recommendation also states that although the risk for listeriosis from deli foods is low, pregnant women and others at risk may want to avoid these foods or thoroughly heat cold cuts before eating.

6. In addition to pregnant women, others at risk for infection with *L. monocytogenes* include neonates, the elderly, immunosuppressed transplant patients, and others with impaired cell-mediated immunity.

7. Listeria monocytogenes possesses several virulence factors. This organism can penetrate intact cells more readily than many other bacteria due to the production of a protein called *internalin*, which induces phagocytosis. Once inside the cell, the organism can avoid the intracellular killing by the combined actions of phospholipases and listeriolysin O. The organisms also produce a protein called Act A which will facilitate cell-to-cell spread of the organism and its progeny.

MICROBIOLOGY CASE 5–6 ANSWERS

1. Many variables come into play when determining the timing and number of blood cultures. These variables include the patient's age, clinical presentation, and the blood culture instrumentation used in the laboratory. Most manufacturers suggest adding 10 mL of blood to each blood culture bottle for adult patients. Special blood culture bottles are available for pediatric patients or for other patients from whom only small volumes of blood can be collected. Special bottles are required for low volumes in order to maintain the appropriate dilution of the blood and the anticoagulants and other additives in the bottles. Statistically, the ability to recover organisms improves with the testing of greater volumes of blood. Studies have shown that 80% of true positives can be detected with one set of blood cultures, 90% are positive with the second, and 99% are positive with the third. Based on these data, a minimum of two sets of blood cultures should be collected, and three sets are considered optimal. Routinely, a set of blood culture bottles consists of one aerobic and one anaerobic bottle. The timing of the collection is again dependent upon the patient's presentation. Whenever possible, blood cultures should be collected before antibiotics are administered. The ideal time for the collection of blood cultures is 30 minutes *before* a fever spike, but this is often impossible to predict. For acute episodes, it is recommended that two sets of cultures be collected at approximately the same time, one set each from two different sites (e.g., opposite arms). In cases of subacute bacterial endocarditis, three sets of blood cultures should be collected on the first day, at least 30 minutes apart.

2. To reduce the chance of contaminating the specimen with organisms from the skin, extremely careful attention must be paid when preparing the site for venipuncture. Preparation should include, at minimum, both an alcohol and an iodine step.

3. Several criteria should be taken into account when trying to determine if a positive blood culture is due to contamination or true bacteremia. These criteria might include the number of bottles that are positive, the length of time it took for the bottles to become positive, the condition of the patient, and whether or not the patient was or is being treated with antimicrobial agents. There are exceptions, but most episodes of true bacteremia will be detected with a positive growth index by 48 hours after incubation. Some exceptions may include slow-growing organisms, low-level bacteremia, or decreased sample volume. Multiple sets of blood culture bottles are collected to increase the chances of recovering the organisms, but this is also helpful since most episodes of true bacteremia will cause two or more of the bottles to give a positive growth index. If one of six bottles becomes positive on the fifth day of incubation and the patient is well and was never on antibiotics, it is likely that that growth is due to contamination. In contrast, if multiple bottles are positive early in incubation and the patient is ill, it is likely to be a true infection.

4. Fred has both bacteremia and septicemia. Bacteremia simply means having bacteria in the blood, while septicemia is the disease (collection of symptoms, syndrome) that the patient experiences as a result of the organisms. The clinical syndrome of septicemia is characterized by fever, chills, malaise, tachycardia, hyperventilation, and toxicity. Bacteremia may be continuous, intermittent, or transient. Transient bacteremia with oral flora may occur after brushing of teeth, for example, but these organisms are usually rapidly cleared from the system in a healthy individual. Intermittent bacteremia may occur when bacteria from an infected body site are sporadically released into the circulatory system. Continuous bacteremia may occur when the organisms are constantly exposed to the circulatory system, as occurs, for example, with endocarditis. The number of positive blood cultures not only can help the physician differentiate between contamination and true bacteremia, but this information may also be useful in determining if the bacteremia is transient or a more serious problem. Since all of Fred's blood cultures were rapidly positive, it is safe to say that he has a true bacteremia, and since he also has a collection of symptoms associated with this bacteremia, he also has the syndrome called *septicemia*.

5. Since the organisms isolated here are gram-positive cocci in chains, one would think of *Streptococcus* and *Enterococcus* spp. The catalase reaction and colony morphology are in keeping with this hypothesis, and the lack of hemolysis rules out some of the *Streptococcus* spp.

6. All things considered, a presumptive identification of *Streptococcus bovis* could be made for the organism isolated from Fred's blood cultures. This organism may be misidentified as a member of the viridans streptococci

group, but the ability to grow in the presence of 40% bile and hydrolyze esculin eliminates that possibility.

7. *S. bovis* is a member of Lancefield group D. *Enterococcus* spp. also possess group D carbohydrates, but the facts that *S. bovis* cannot grow in 6.5% NaCl and is PYR negative differentiate it from the *Enterococcus* spp.

8. More definitive identification of streptococci and other gram-positive cocci may also be accomplished with a number of commercially available kits or automated or semiautomated identification systems. (A few examples include Vitek GPI, API Rapid Strep, RapID STR, and MicroScan Pos ID panel.)

9. There is a striking association between *S. bovis* bacteremia and colon cancer. This organism is also capable of causing endocarditis, and this may also have occurred as a secondary complication in this patient. Given Fred's history and the bacteremia with *S. bovis*, colon cancer would certainly be among the conditions the physician would be considering. Fred has a complex presentation. With the history of alcohol and tobacco use, it is also possible (expected) that signs of liver disease and lung damage would be demonstrated in his clinical laboratory findings.

MICROBIOLOGY CASE 5–7 ANSWERS

1. Given Bobby's age and history, the cerebrospinal fluid (CSF) parameters, Gram's stain, and colony characteristics, *Haemophilus influenzae* is most likely causing his infection.

2. Members of this genus require growth factors found in blood (Haemophilus means "blood loving"). Some organisms in this genus have a requirement for X factor, which is a collection of heat-stable compounds found in iron-containing pigments like hemin. Most members of this genus require V factor or nicotinamide adenine dinucleotide (NAD). Both X and V factors are found in sheep RBC used in the preparation of the routine BAP. However, the blood also contains an NADase that breaks down the V factor in the plate preventing organisms that require this factor from growing on a routine BAP. In the preparation of CHOC agar, the blood is heated by addition to the molten agar. The heating lyses the RBC, releases the X and V factors, and inactivates the enzymes that hydrolyze the NAD. As a result, CHOC agar is commonly used for the recovery of *Haemophilus* spp. in the clinical laboratory. *Haemophilus* spp. that require NAD will also exhibit a satelliting phenomenon around *Staphylococcus aureus*. The *S. aureus* organisms lyse the RBC and inactivate the enzymes that hydrolyze the NAD. Determining if *Haemophilus* spp. require X factor, V factor, or both can be helpful in speciating these organisms.

3. It is possible to test an organism's requirement for X and V factor using several methods:

    a. One method uses filter paper disks or strips containing X, V, and both X&V. When performing this test, it is important to use a Mueller-Hinton agar plate or other minimal media that is lacking both factors.

Using sterile saline as diluent, a suspension of the organism is prepared with a turbidity equivalent to a 0.5 McFarland standard. The suspension is used to inoculate a lawn of organism on the plate, and the disks are placed on the plate. After overnight incubation, the plate is examined for growth around the disks. If an organism grows only around the X&V disk, it requires both factors. If an organism grows around one of the single-factor disks (and the X&V disk), it requires that factor. It is possible to omit the X&V-factor disk if the individual factor disks are placed 3 to 5 mm apart on the plate. This requires more careful reading, but if growth is present only between the disks, it indicates that the organism requires both factors. If the organism grows all the way around a single-factor disk, it indicates that it requires that single factor.

b. Commercially available quad plates are also convenient. These plates have four sections; one each that contains X, V, both X&V, and both X&V plus horse blood. Each section of the plate is inoculated lightly with the organism, and the plate is incubated overnight. The observation of growth in the various quadrants allows the laboratory scientist to determine the growth requirements of the organism being tested. The observation of hemolysis in the horse blood is also helpful for speciation.

c. As mentioned previously, most *Haemophilus* spp. will demonstrate satelliting around an *S. aureus* streak on BAP, indicating the requirement for V factor. In conjunction with this, it will be necessary to determine if the organism requires X factor. The requirement for X factor can be determined using the delta-aminolevulinic acid (ALA) test, or porphyrin test. Organisms that require X factor (heme) do so because they lack an enzyme that would allow them to produce the factor from its precursors. In this test, the delta-aminolevulinic acid substrate is inoculated with the organism and the production of porphyrin intermediaries is detected using UV light or Kovac's reagent after 4 to 24 hours' incubation. If the organism is positive in this test, it indicates that it can produce porphyrin (and eventually heme) and therefore would *not* require X factor. A negative ALA test indicates that the organism requires X factor.

4. The extremely elevated protein, decreased glucose, and extremely elevated WBC in this CSF are consistent with bacterial meningitis. The decreased glucose is due to the fact that the organisms will metabolize glucose and decrease the level of this analyte in the fluid. The WBC count is increased due to the immune system response to the invading organisms, and the protein is elevated due to the presence of protein in the actual organisms. These parameters are not consistent with other types of meningitis (fungal or viral).

5. In children between 3 months and 18 years of age, *Neisseria meningitidis* and *Streptococcus pneumoniae* are common pathogens of bacterial meningitis.

6. Direct CSF latex agglutination testing is available for some common causes of bacterial meningitis including *H. influenzae* type b, *Streptococcus pneumoniae, Neisseria meningitidis*, and *Streptococcus agalactiae* (common in neonates). This testing uses latex particles that are coated with specific antibodies directed against the capsular antigen of the organism. This testing should be used with caution, since the sensitivity is much lower than culture. A positive test is very helpful in confirming the suspicion of a particular pathogen based on the Gram's stain, the age of the patient, and so on, but a negative result should be interpreted with caution: A negative test does not necessarily mean that the patient does not have meningitis. In the case of a negative latex test, the amount of antigen (organism) may be below the level of detection of the system, or the patient may have meningitis caused by a type of *H. influenzae* other than b, a non-typeable strain of *H. influenzae*, or a completely different organism not included in the kit. Given these caveats, this testing is appropriate when the patient has been treated with antibiotics before the collection of the CSF specimen. In this situation, the culture would be compromised due to the antibiotics, although the nonviable organisms may still be present in great enough numbers to yield a positive latex agglutination test.

7. A very effective vaccine is available for *H. influenzae* type b, and this vaccine is part of the recommended childhood immunization schedule. Since the patient described in this case was not immunized, he was susceptible to infection with this organism. Before the immunization initiative, this pathogen was the number one cause of meningitis in children under 5 years of age. As a result of widespread immunization, meningitis caused by *H. influenzae* type b has declined by 95%. In fact, the rate of meningitis cases in general has declined significantly because this pathogen was responsible for such a large portion of the cases of meningitis. Along with immunization, rifampin prophylaxis of disease contacts is also effective in preventing the spread of this infection.

MICROBIOLOGY CASE 5–8 ANSWERS

1. The organism causing these surgical wound infections is *Staphylococcus aureus*. Based on the resistance to oxacillin, it can be described further as a methicillin-resistant *S. aureus* (MRSA). MRSA can be a significant epidemiological problem in hospitals, long-term care facilities, and other health care institutions. The prevalence of MRSA in the United States varies by region. The average is in the range of 10% to 15% but can vary from 5% to 20% of *S. aureus* isolated. Approximately 20% to 30% of the healthy population carries *S. aureus* on their skin or in the nares, and health care providers (physicians, nurses, laboratory workers, ward attendants) often have an even higher carriage rate with this organism.

2. *S. aureus* has many characteristic reactions that are very helpful in its identification. Along with the beta-hemolysis and the coagulase-positive reaction, *S. aureus* is mannitol positive (bright yellow colonies on mannitol salt

agar). Rapid latex agglutination tests are also available for the identification of *S. aureus*. These latex agglutination tests often take advantage of the fact that *S. aureus* produces a protein that binds nonspecifically to the Fc portion of antibody molecules. The manufacturers bind the antibodies to latex beads, making it easier to observe the agglutination. Another characteristic that is sometimes useful is the fact that the organism possess a DNAse. Several methods are available that can determine this activity.

3. To accurately determine resistance to oxacillin, antimicrobial susceptibility testing with *S. aureus* should be performed in an increased sodium chloride environment, or incubation should occur at 30°C. The exact concentration of sodium chloride is dependent upon the assay method employed and can vary from 2% to 5%. Most commercially prepared antimicrobial susceptibility testing methods take this into consideration and are prepared with an appropriate sodium chloride concentration.

4. Methicillin-resistant *S. aureus* is effectively treated with vancomycin.

5. Nosocomial infections are infections acquired in a hospital or institutional setting. Generally, if an infection occurs 48 to 72 hours after a patient has been admitted to a hospital or institution, it may be considered a nosocomial infection. It is important to point out, however, that due to extended incubation periods for some types of infections a nosocomial infection may not become apparent until after the patient has been discharged. For example, a patient may be exposed to chickenpox while in the hospital, but due to the 7- to 10-day incubation period of the virus, symptoms of the infection may not be obvious until the patient is at home.

6. Hand washing is the single most effective way to prevent the spread of infection.

7. Many techniques are useful in epidemiological investigations to determine if the same or different strains of organism are at the root of an outbreak or proposed outbreak. Historically, resistance phenotyping, bacteriophage typing, immunoserology, and serotyping were of some value in determining strain relatedness. More recently, electrophoretic protein typing, multilocus enzyme electrophoresis, and genetic techniques like plasmid analysis, restriction endonuclease analysis of chromosomal DNA, restriction fragment length polymorphisms, ribotyping, and nucleic acid sequence analysis have been employed to determine strain identity or relatedness.

MICROBIOLOGY CASE 5–9 ANSWERS

1. The description of the parasite, in particular the "face-like" appearance, along with the history and physical presentation leads to *Giardia lamblia*.

2. Giardiasis is sometimes called "beaver fever," since beaver and other mammals can act as a reservoir for the pathogen. The pathogen may be encountered in untreated water from streams and rivers that have been contaminated with animal or human feces. The organism is most often acquired through contaminated water, but food-borne and person-to-person trans-

mission have also been reported. Maria probably acquired the disease from handling the animals or from the water during her fieldwork.

3. The centrally located dark bands are called *axonemes*.

4. Before the ova and parasite evaluation are performed, other significant intestinal parasites suspected might be *Entamoeba histolytica, Dientamoeba fragilis,* and *Blastocystis hominis,* although the pathogenicity of *B. hominis* remains controversial. Due to the probable zoonotic (animal-transmitted) nature of Maria's disease, *Cryptosporidium parvum* and even *Isospora belli* might also be suspect, although very severe disease caused by these organisms is more likely in an immunocompromised host.

5. Many patients shed parasite eggs or cysts intermittently, and therefore a single stool specimen may not be sufficient to isolate the pathogen. A series of three specimens should be collected over a 7- to 10-day period, and the specimen collection should be spaced a day or two apart.

6. Both techniques are suggested because, while one technique is more sensitive (in general), the other provides more structural detail. Concentration techniques are employed to remove much of the fecal debris and concentrate the parasites in a smaller volume. Cysts, larvae, and some ova can be detected in concentrates, but trophozoites and operculated ova do not concentrate well. Trophozoites are much more likely to be seen in permanently stained smears, and these preparations are more useful for the detection of nuclear detail and internal structures of the organisms. Commonly used permanent stains include trichrome and iron hematoxylin.

7. *Clostridium difficile* disease, or *C. difficile*-associated pseduomembranous colitis, is caused by *C. difficile* toxin. *C. difficile* disease can be a serious complication of other medical treatment (see answer 8) as well as a very serious nosocomial and epidemiological problem. This is especially true with elderly patients and in extended-care facilities.

8. *C. difficile*-associated pseudomembranous colitis is also sometimes called *antibiotic-associated pseduomembranous colitis* because the disease often occurs after 5 to 10 days of antibiotic therapy. It is important to note, however, that cases have been reported after only 1 day of therapy or as late as 10 weeks after therapy. The fact that Maria took antibiotics may have triggered the physician's suspicion.

9. The classic, "gold standard" *C. difficile* toxin assay is a cytotoxicity assay in which the effects of the toxin are observed on a monolayer (single layer) of cells in culture. The stool specimen is filtered, diluted, and added to the medium above the monolayer with and without antitoxin (toxin-neutralizing antibody). The cells are observed at 24 and 48 hours for any signs of damage, or cytopathic effect (CPE). Since there may be other substances in feces that are toxic to the cells in this assay, it is necessary to confirm that the effects are indeed caused by the toxin. If CPE is noted in a well with sample and not noted in the well with sample plus antitoxin, the specimen is considered a true-positive. If a specimen demonstrates CPE in the presence of the antitoxin, it is considered a false-positive. Enzyme-linked

immunosorbent assay (ELISA) kits are also available for the detection of *C. difficile* toxin, but the kits are generally not as sensitive as the cytotoxicity assay.

10. The disease is caused by the toxin, not merely by the presence of the organism. It is necessary to demonstrate the presence of the toxin, since many individuals may carry the organisms in very low numbers, or individuals may carry nonpathogenic (toxin-negative) strains. It is not until the normal microbial balance in the colon is disrupted (by antibiotics or other chemotherapeutic agents) that the toxin-producing organisms begin to cause disease.

MICROBIOLOGY CASE 5–10 ANSWERS

1. *Enterobacter cloacae* is most likely the organism causing Elmer's infection.

2. Along with the common Gram's stain reaction of gram-negative bacilli, members of the family *Enterobacteriaceae* are also all glucose positive, nitrate reductase positive, and oxidase negative.

3. When trying to identify organisms in the family *Enterobacteriaceae*, it is helpful to pick out some key characteristics to narrow down the search. These key characteristics include VP-positive, H_2S-positive, motility, and the phenylalanine deaminase (PAD)-positive groups. The Voges-Proskauer (VP)-positive organisms include the *Klebsiella, Enterobacter, Hafnia*, and *Serratia* spp. The H_2S-positive organisms include *Salmonella, Proteus*, and *Edwardsiella* spp., and *Citrobacter freundii*. The *non*-motile (at 35°C) organisms include *Shigella, Klebsiella*, and *Yersinia* spp. The PAD-positive organisms include *Proteus* and *Providencia* spp. and *Morganella morganii*.

4. Because this organism is VP positive, it is in the KES group. Given the fact that this organism is motile, the *Klebsiella* spp. can be ruled out. Also, since the organism is DNase negative, the *Serratia* spp. can be ruled out, leaving the *Enterobacter* spp.

5. After the genus *Enterobacter* is identified, the helpful biochemical reactions for speciation include lysine and ornithine decarboxylase, arginine dihydrolase, and sorbitol.

6. Indole tests determine if an organism has the enzyme tryptophanase. Since indole is one of the degradation products from the metabolism of tryptophan, this amino acid must be present in the growth media used for indole tests.

7. The nitrate reductase test determines if an organism can convert nitrate to nitrite. To make the determination, the organism is grown in the nitrate broth, and after sufficient growth is obtained, reagent A (alpha-naphthylamine in acetic acid) and reagent B (sulfanilic acid in acetic acid) are added. If nitrate has been converted to nitrite, a red color develops after the addition of the reagents. If no color forms, no nitrite is present. The absence of nitrite could be due to the fact that the organism is unable to convert nitrate to nitrite, *or* it could be due to the fact that the organism has

further converted the nitrite to nitrogen gas or other gaseous nitrogen compounds. Zinc dust must be added when a colorless reaction is seen in order to differentiate between these two possibilities. When the organism cannot make the reductase enzyme, the addition of the zinc dust converts the remaining nitrate to nitrite, and a pink color results (pink after zinc confirms a negative result). True positive reactions remain colorless after the addition of zinc dust.

8. The methyl red (MR) and Voges-Proskauer (VP) tests determine the end products that are produced as a result of glucose fermentation. If large quantities of mixed acid end products are produced, the organism is positive in the MR test. Methyl red is a pH indicator that will appear red below pH 4.4. If neutral end products (acetoin) are produced, the organism is positive in the VP test. A red color is formed when 40% KOH is combined with acetoin, and this color is intensified by the addition of alpha-naphthol.

9. Because this organism is lactose positive, it would most likely appear as a pink colony on MAC. It is important to note, however, that the rapidity with which colonies of this organism turn pink on MAC is dependent on the presence of the beta-galactoside permease enzyme. This enzyme allows the lactose to be transported into the cell for metabolism.

10.   a. The carbohydrates present in triple-sugar iron (TSI) agar include glucose, lactose, and sucrose. The concentration of lactose and sucrose is 10 times greater than the concentration of glucose in this medium. Glucose-fermenting organisms will initially (within 8 to 12 hours) use glucose as a carbohydrate source and acidify the entire medium in a TSI. Due to the relatively small amount of glucose present, this carbohydrate is quickly exhausted. When glucose has been used, the butt portion of the slant will remain acidic (yellow) for the remainder of the incubation period (unless the organism is H_2S positive, in which case, a black precipitate will be formed, obscuring the color of the butt). When glucose has been exhausted, the organisms that have the ability to do so will switch to one of the other carbohydrate sources (glucose effect). Use of lactose and/or sucrose will keep the slant portion of the TSI acidic.

   If an organism does *not* have the ability to use lactose or sucrose, when the glucose is exhausted, the organisms will be forced to use protein as an energy source via oxidative degradation of the amino acids. This can only occur in the slant since oxygen is required. The end products of this metabolism result in a neutralization of the slant (red color) after 18 to 24 hours incubation. Therefore, a red slant indicates that the organisms were not able to use lactose or sucrose.

   b. Since the organism described is A/A on TSI and colorless on MAC, it can be concluded that the organism is glucose positive (acid butt on TSI), lactose negative (colorless on MAC), and sucrose positive (acid slant on TSI).

ANSWERS FOR CHAPTER 6, URINALYSIS CASES

URINALYSIS CASE 6–1 ANSWERS

1. The abnormal macroscopic findings are appearance, cloudy; protein, 1+(30 mg/dL) (sulfosalicylic acid [SSA], 1+); blood, 1+; nitrite, positive; leukocyte esterase, 2+. The abnormal microscopic findings are white blood cells (WBCs), 40 to 60/high-power field (HPF) (2 to 4 clumps/HPF); casts, 3 to 6 WBC/low-power field (LPF), 0 to 2 granular/LPF; 0 to 1 bacterial/LPF. Discrepant results: none.

2. The presence of renal epithelial cells and casts are consistent with an upper urinary tract infection. Renal epithelial cells line various parts of the nephron and indicate a renal origin. They are usually reported as renal tubular epithelial, although they can be divided into convoluted renal tubular cells from the proximal and distal convoluted tubules and collecting duct cells from the collecting ducts. Rare renal epithelial cells indicate only normal sloughing off and replacement of old cells, but in greater numbers, they may point to more significant damage to the tubules and collecting ducts. Casts are also formed only in the renal tubules (distal convoluted tubule and collecting duct); therefore, their presence often signifies renal involvement.

3. a. The urinalysis results are indicative of acute pyelonephritis.

   b. Acute pyelonephritis is characterized by mild proteinuria (<1 g/d); leukocyte esterase +/±; nitrite +/±; increased WBCs; bacteria; WBC, granular, renal cell, and waxy casts; red blood cells (RBCs) and renal epithelial cells. Chronic pyelonephritis is differentiated by moderate proteinuria (<2.5 g/d); leukocyte esterase ±; increased WBCs; granular, waxy, and broad casts; and few WBC and renal cell casts. The history of recurrent infections is the hallmark of chronic pyelonephritis.

4. Pyuria is associated with neutrophils, that is, polymorphonuclear neutrophils (PMNs).

5. Leukocyte casts are pathognomic of this disease, although they may be found in other conditions. The WBCs in WBC casts can be from the glomeruli or tubules. If they are glomerular in origin (glomerulonephritis), red cells casts would also be present and in larger numbers than leukocyte casts. A tubular source (pyelonephritis) would have bacteria along with the leukocyte casts. In this patient the urinalysis and related information point to a tubular source, that is, pyelonephritis.

6. Two mechanisms leading to acute pyelonephritis are (a) ascending pyelonephritis—bacteria moving up the urinary tract—that is cystitis (bladder), to the kidney and (b) hematogenous pyelonephritis—bacteria in the circulatory tract settling in the kidney.

7. Reflex testing would include a urine culture and sensitivity. *Escherichia coli* is the most common pathogen, although *Proteus, Klebsiella, Enterobacter,* and *Pseudomonas* spp. are also frequently identified causes of pyelonephritis.

8. The treatment is a suitable antibiotic. The most frequently used antibiotics are furidantin, amoxicillin, cephalosporins, sulfisoxazole/trimethoprim, and sulfa drugs for 10 to 14 days. Patients must be cautioned to complete the entire course of antibiotics even if the symptoms have subsided and they are feeling better.

9. Pyelonephritis is most often caused by untreated cystitis when the bacteria continue to migrate up the urinary tract through the ureters and finally to the kidney (pyelonephritis). Catherization, diabetes mellitus, pregnancy, and urinary obstruction increase the risk for acute pyelonephritis. Other people prone to pyelonephritis are individuals with cancer or acquired immune deficiency syndrome (AIDS) (immunocompromised patients), recurrent cystitis, benign prostate hyperplasia, and structural abnormalities (vesicoureteric reflux—persistent backflow of the urine from the bladder into the ureters).

10. Most patients with acute pyelonephritis recover without complications. Complications can include recurrence of pyelonephritis (chronic pyelonephritis), sepsis, and in rare cases acute renal failure. Acute pyelonephritis should be treated carefully and completely especially in elderly patients, who are more likely to have severe cases and recurrent infections.

URINALYSIS CASE 6–2 ANSWERS

1. The abnormal macroscopic urinalysis results are color, red; appearance, cloudy; protein, 3+ (100 mg/dL) (SSA:2+); and blood, 2+. The abnormal microscopic results are RBCs, 30 to 60/HPF; casts, 0 to 3 RBC/LPF, 0 to 1 hemoglobin/LPF, and 1 to 3 granular/LPF. Discrepant results: none.

2. The urinalysis is indicative of acute glomerulonephritis (AGN). AGN onset is usually acute, and symptoms include fever, oliguria, malaise, edema, hematuria, and proteinuria. Poststreptococcal glomerulonephritis occurs 1 to 2 weeks after inadequate or nontreatment of a streptococcal throat infection, as in this case.

3. Erythrocytes (RBCs)and erythrocyte and hemoglobin casts are pathognomic of AGN. Erythrocyte and hemoglobin casts are indicative of renal disease of glomerular origin (glomerulonephritis), although tubular damage may result in the formation of these casts. Erythrocyte casts are most commonly associated with glomerulopnephritis.

4. Dysmorphic RBCs usually indicate glomerular damage. The RBCs have been in the ultrafiltrate (urine) from the glomerulus to the urethra; therefore, they have been exposed to a hypertonic environment for a longer period of time than those entering lower in the urinary tract, that is, the bladder. This may result in damage to the erythrocyte membrane and dysmorphic erythrocytes.

5. Reagent strip protein is more sensitive and specific for albumin and may not measure globulins, Bence Jones protein, or Tamm-Horsfall glycoproteins. SSA will precipitate most proteins including albumin, glycoprotein,

and globulins. Multistix reagent strips are sensitive to 15 to 30 mg/dL, Chemstrip reagent strips are sensitive to 6 mg/dL, and SSA is sensitive to 5 to 10 mg/dL.

6. The 24-hour protein is consistent with AGN: usually mild (<1 g/24h), but it can reach nephrotic levels (>3.5 g/24h). The level of proteinuria in glomerulonephritis varies with the level of glomerular damage, and normally in AGN only mild proteinuria is noted.

7. The causative agent is group A beta-hemolytic streptococci. Specific strains of group A beta-strep are nephritogenic, especially types 1, 4, and 12, which have the M protein in their cell walls. AGN is caused by the formation of immune complexes including antibodies and streptococcal antigens. This stimulates proliferation of endothelial and mesangial cells as well as leukocytic (neutrophils and monocytes) infiltration and the glomeruli become hypercellular. Fibrin deposits within the capillary lumina can also be detected. Poststreptococcal glomerulonephritis is the most common type of GN, with an incidence of <20/100,000, usually found in children 2 to 12 years old.

8. Other causes for AGN:
   a. Acute postinfectious glomerulonephritis
      i. Other gram-positives: *Streptococcus viridans, Staphylococcus aureus*
      ii. Gram-negatives: *Klebsiella pneumoniae, Salmonella typhus*
      iii. Viral: hepatitis B, cytomegalovirus, Epstein-Barr virus, and human immunodeficiency virus
      iv. Parasites: plasmodia, toxoplasma
   b. Immunoglobulin A (IgA) (±IgG) deposition
      i. Systemic lupus erythematosus
      ii. IgA nephropathy
      iii. Henoch-Schönlein purpura
   c. Concurrent infection
      i. Bacterial endocarditis
      ii. Shunt nephritis
      iii. Visceral abscess
   d. Autoimmune disease
   e. Membranoproliferative glomerulonephritis

9. Yes, serum urea nitrogen (BUN) and creatinine are elevated in AGN due to a decreased glomerular filtration rate.

10. Yes, the BUN/creatinine (BUN/CR) ratio is 17.5 (the BUN divided by the CR 28 ÷ 1.6), with elevated BUN and CR, which indicates renal disease. A normal BUN/CR ratio is between 1:10 and 1:20, and a normal ratio with elevated BUN and CR indicates renal disease. Lower ratios are found in acute tubular necrosis (ATN), low protein intake, starvation, or severe liver disease. High ratios with normal CR are associated with prerenal azotemia, high protein

intake, and catabolic tissue breakdown. High ratios with elevated CR suggest postrenal obstruction or prerenal azotemia with renal disease.

11. Creatinine clearance performed on a 24-hour urine specimen and a serum sample provides useful information. Creatinine clearance would be decreased due to the decrease in glomerular filtration rate.

12. The ASO titer is increased in the two sequelae of group A streptococcal infection: AGN and rheumatic fever. Anti-DNAse B is produced by group A streptococci and can be detected earlier than ASO. It is the most specific test for detecting an antecedent group A strep infection, AGN, and rheumatic fever. C-3 is decreased in glomerulonephritis due to its increased catabolism in the circulating immune complexes.

13. Poststreptococcal glomerulonephritis usually resolves spontaneously after a few weeks or months. Recovery is complete in 90% of patients (especially children), but in 5% to 10%, the disease progresses to chronic glomerulonephritis.

URINALYSIS CASE 6–3 ANSWERS

1. The abnormal macroscopic urinalysis results are appearance, cloudy/frothy; and protein, 3+. The abnormal microscopic results are casts, 0 to 1 renal tubular epithelial/LPF; 0 to 1 granular/LPF; 0 to 1 waxy/LPF; and 0 to1 fatty/LPF; occasional oval fat bodies. Discrepant results: none.

2. Bonnie's urinalysis is consistent with nephrotic syndrome.

3. The basic defect is damage to the glomerular basement membrane in the renal nephron, which results in increased permeability of the glomerulus. The damage in some types of nephrotic syndrome is caused by the deposits of immune complexes (antigen–antibody) in the basement membrane. Changes in the electrical charges in the basal lamina and podocytes of the basement membrane allow higher molecular weight molecules, proteins and lipids, into the glomerular filtrate. Nephrotic syndrome is not actually a disease but a condition based on a combination of signs and symptoms. Brunzel (1994, p. 148) defines it as "a complication of numerous diseases characterized by the presentation of proteinuria, hypoalbuminuria, hyperlipidemia, lipiduria and generalized edema."

4. Marked proteinuria and lipiduria (oval fat bodies and fatty casts) are hallmarks of nephrotic syndrome. As mentioned in question 3, proteins and lipids are found in the urine due to changes in the basement membrane of the glomeruli caused by deposits of immune complexes on the cells of the basement membrane.

5. a. The presence of oval fat bodies can be confirmed using a lipid stain, e.g., Sudan III or oil red O. The fat droplets are very refractile and vary in size. Oval fat bodies with cholesterol also exhibit the characteristic Maltese Cross pattern with polarized light.

   b. Oval fat bodies are degenerating or necrotic renal tubular cells with inclusions of fat or lipids.

6. The frothy urine is consistent with proteinuria and may be the first sign of nephrotic syndrome. Moderate-to-heavy proteinuria will alter the surface tension of the urine, causing a white foam to be produced when the urine is poured or agitated. It is thick and lasts longer than other "normal" foam.

7. a. Primary: glomerulonephritis
    b. Secondary:
        i. Diabetes mellitus
        ii. Lupus erythematosus
        iii. Multiple myeloma
        iv. Acquired immune deficiency syndrome
        v. Autoimmune disorders
        vi. Infections
        vii. Congenital heart disease
        viii. Toxins
        ix. Severe allergic disorders
        x. Medications (e.g., penicillamine, probenecid, captopril)

8. Risk factors for nephrotic syndrome
    a. Family history of nephrotic syndrome (primary cause)
    b. Pregnancy
    c. Exposure to chemical toxins
    d. Congestive heart failure
    e. Lymphomas
    f. Drug addiction
    g. Immunosuppression (drugs or disease)

9. Nephrotic syndrome is characterized by hypoalbuminemia and hyperlipidemia (elevated cholesterol). (See answers to questions 3 and 5.) Hyperlipidemia is inversely proportional to the albumin concentration: The lower the albumin levels fall, the higher the lipid values. Liver synthesis of all proteins increases to compensate for the increased loss of protein in the urine, and large proteins (haptoglobin), which are retained, are increased in the blood. Hypoalbuminemia stimulates the liver to synthesize low-density lipoproteins (LDL) and very-low-density lipoproteins (VLDLs). The minimally increased BUN and creatinine are indicative of slightly decreased renal function.

10. Creatinine clearance, 24-hour urine volume, and 24-hour urine protein could be performed. The creatinine clearance would be normal or slightly decreased in nephrotic syndrome. The 24-hour urine volume is decreased, sometimes to 20% of normal. The 24-hour urine protein is usually increased to greater than 3.5 g/d.

11. The edema is caused by the hypoalbuminemia, which leads to reduced plasma oncotic pressure. The reduced oncotic pressure allows fluids to leak from blood vessels to the interstitial spaces, resulting in edema. Abnormal salt and water retention also contribute to the edema.

12. The patient's protein electrophoresis would be characterized by a marked increase in alpha$_2$- and beta-globulins, and a marked decrease in albumin and gamma-globulins, especially IgG.

13. The protein selectivity index reflects the ability of the glomerulus to hold back larger proteins but allow smaller proteins like albumin into the glomerular filtrate. It is calculated as the IgG/albumin clearance ratio. The index is inversely proportional to the selectivity: An index of 0.16 indicates a high selectivity (mostly albumin), and an index of 0.30 suggests poor selectivity (nonselective proteinuria). Poor selectivity indicates that the glomeruli are allowing all proteins through regardless of size, larger globulins as well as albumin. The protein selectivity index can give the physician an idea of how much damage has been done to the glomeruli—the lower the selectivity, the more damage has been done.

14. Nephrotic syndrome can lead to venous and arterial thrombus, increased susceptibility to infections, and abnormal lipid metabolism (vascular disease). Other complications include chronic kidney disease leading to renal failure.

URINALYSIS CASE 6–4 ANSWERS

1. The abnormal macroscopic findings (day 1/day 2) are appearance, cloudy/cloudy; nitrite, pos/pos; and leukocyte esterase, 2+/2+. Abnormal microscopic results (day 2) are WBCs, 25 to 40/HPF; and bacteria, moderate. Discrepant results: None.

2. a. The absence of casts indicates a lower urinary tract infection.
   b. Casts are the primary indicator of a renal problem because they are formed *only* in the kidney, primarily in the distal convoluted tubule and collecting duct.

3. This young woman has cystitis. Infections in the lower urinary tract, most commonly cystitis, are characterized by pyuria (increased WBCs) and the absence of casts (see answer to question 2).

4. a. No, it would not change the diagnosis, because false-negative leukocyte esterase and nitrite results are possible. False-negative leukocyte esterase can be caused by the following:
      i. Low numbers of WBCs. Leukocyte esterase (L.E.) detects 10 to 25 WBCs/μL. The number of WBCs may be increased but not high enough to produce a positive result.
      ii. WBCs present which are not granulocytes and do not produce leukocyte esterase.
      iii. Increased glucose, protein, and specific gravity, which decrease the sensitivity of the L.E. reaction and can result in a false-negative result.
   b. False-negative nitrite reaction can be caused by the following:
      i. Infection by bacteria that do *not* reduce nitrate, that is, are gram-positive bacteria.

       ii. Bacteria not being present in the bladder for a sufficient length of time to allow nitrate reduction. In urinary tract infections, frequency of urination may not allow sufficient time for nitrate reduction.

       iii. A patient with a nitrate-deficient diet not producing enough nitrate to result in a positive nitrite reaction.

5. Increased numbers of transitional epithelial cells are sloughed off from the renal calyces, renal pelves, ureters, bladder, and urethra (of males) during infection/ inflammation.

6. Cystitis is usually caused by fecal flora: *Escherichia coli* (75% to 95%), *Klebsiella* sp. (5%), *Proteus, Pseudomonas,* spp., and others. A colony-forming unit count of 100,000 mL is usually considered diagnostic for an infection.

7. Cranberry juice reduces pyuria and bacteriuria by reducing *E. coli* adherence to cells. The acidity of the juice also sets up a less favorable environment for bacterial growth. Vitamin C supplements also acidify the urine.

8. Increased urine production will facilitate the excretion of bacteria from the bladder, because increased urine flow from the bladder helps to wash bacteria out of the bladder and urethra. Bacteria move up the urinary tract from the urethra (urethritis) to the bladder (cystitis) and if untreated to the kidney (pyelonephritis).

9. Women have shorter urethras, providing the bacteria easier access to the bladder. Three other reasons include

   a. Increased hormone levels appear to enhance adherence of the bacteria to the mucosa

   b. During sexual intercourse, bacteria on the external genitalia may be pushed up the urethra to the bladder

   c. Women do not have a prostate gland and therefore do not produce prostatic fluid, which inhibits the growth of bacteria.

10. Diabetes, calculi (kidney stones), prostatic hyperplasia, pregnancy, and catherization are associated with an increased incidence of cystitis. It is thought pregnant women are more prone to cystitis because of hormone changes and possible changes in position of the kidney during pregnancy.

URINALYSIS CASE 6–5 ANSWERS

1. The abnormal macroscopic and microscopic results are color, brown; protein, 1+; casts, 0 to 1 granular/LPF. Discrepant results: blood, 3+; and RBCs, 0 to 1/HPF.

2. Hemoglobinuria and myoglobinuria produce positive reactions with the blood reagent strip and negative microscopics (no RBCs in the sediment).

3.   a. Hematuria
     i. Transfusion reaction
     ii. Hemolytic anemia
     iii. Strenuous exercise

      iv. Drugs, e.g., anticoagulants

      v. Severe burns

      vi. Infections

      vii. Paroxysmal nocturnal hemoglobinuria

    b. Myoglobinuria (rhabdomyolysis)

      i. Increased muscular activity, i.e., sports

      ii. Muscle injury, i.e., trauma (crush injuries), burns

      iii. Infections, bacterial and viral

      iv. Drugs, e.g., alcohol, opiates, cocaine

      v. Toxins, e.g., ethanol, ethylene glycol, isopropyl alcohol

      vi. Metabolic disorders, e.g., diabetic ketoacidosis, hyponatremia, hypokalemia

4. The most probable cause is myoglobinuria (rhabdomyolysis) due to crush injuries.

5. Rhabdomylosis is an acute, sometimes fatal disease caused by the release of muscle cell contents into circulation. Enzymes including creatine kinase, aspartate aminotransferase, lactate dehydrogenase, and aldolase; myoglobin; and electrolytes are released into the blood stream. Rhabdomyolysis may result in myoglobinuria, which can lead to acute renal failure. Myoglobin may obstruct renal tubules, causing renal damage, and myoglobin also breaks down into toxic compounds, which can also lead to renal failure.

6. The simplest screening test is solubility in ammonium sulfate. In 80% ammonium sulfate (2.8 g/5 mL of urine), hemoglobin precipitates out of solution, but myoglobin will remain in solution. Add ammonium sulfate, allow the solution to react for 3 minutes, and filter. If the reactant was myoglobin, the filtrate remains positive for blood; if it was hemoglobin, it will be negative because the hemoglobin has precipitated out.

7. The excretion of large quantities of myoglobin results in kidney damage and can lead to acute tubular necrosis.

8. Creatine kinase (CK) and lactate dehydrogenase are elevated in muscle injury. CK levels rise 2 to 12 hours after injury, peak in 1 to 3 days, and return to normal within 3 to 5 days. Lactate dehydrogenase is also elevated in muscle injuries, but the levels are not as high as CK. In hemoglobinuria, CK is usually less than 10 times the upper reference limit, whereas in myoglobinuria, the CK can be greater than 40 times the reference limit.

9. Serum and urine myoglobin, uric acid, and potassium are elevated in rhabdomyolysis (an acute, sometimes fatal disease characterized by the destruction of muscle tissue). Myoglobin immunoassays are available, although not performed routinely in most clinical laboratories. The slow clearance of CK from the plasma results in higher CK levels for a longer period of time than myoglobin. Serum potassium may be very high due to the release of potassium from the injured cells into the blood stream.

URINALYSIS CASE 6–6 ANSWERS

1. The abnormal macroscopic results are protein, trace (SSA = trace) 5 to 20 mg/dL; blood, 1+; leukocyte esterase, trace; urobilinogen, 4 mg/dL. The abnormal microscopic results are 10 to 20 WBCs/HPF; 30 to 40 RBCs/HPF; casts, 10 to 20 hyaline/LPF; 10 to 15 granular/LPF. Discrepant results: none.

2. The following conditions could manifest some or all of the abnormal results identified in question 1:
   a. Renal disease, e.g., glomerulonephritis: protein, blood, WBCs, and casts infection.
   b. Calculi
   c. Tumor
   d. Lesions
   e. Drugs, e.g., anticoagulants
   f. Bleeding disorders
   g. Severe physical exercise (athletic pseudonephritis)

3. No, Tammy should not be unduly alarmed at the results. Her physician can probably rule out a number of possibilities with a physical examination and medical history.

4. Severe physical exercise was probably responsible for the abnormal urinalysis results. A urinalysis indicating 25 to 40 hyaline or granular casts per low-power field can be seen in athletic pseudonephritis. The granules in the granular casts in nonpathogical conditions appear to be lysosomes excreted by the renal tubular cells, which are increased during periods of stress or exercise.

5. In pathological conditions such as glomerulonephritis and pyelonephritis, the granular casts are formed by the disintegration of cellular casts and tubule cells or protein filtered by the glomerulus.

6. A repeat urinalysis after a period of rest can be used to rule out any renal problems. A repeat urinalysis after 24 to 28 hours will most likely be normal (negative protein and casts).

7. a. Granular casts in pathological conditions will be accompanied by cellular casts (RBC, WBC, or renal tubular).
   b. In nonpathological conditions, the sediment will consist of mainly hyaline and granular casts.

URINALYSIS CASE 6–7 ANSWERS

1. The abnormal/discrepant result is the negative blood on the reagent strip and 25 to 30 RBCs in the sediment.

2. The technologist should first repeat the urinalysis on the original specimen if enough urine is available. The name and hospital number on the original specimen container and the number on the centrifuge tube should be verified *before* repeating the sediment. If the quantity is not sufficient, a new specimen should be requested.

3. A new specimen should be requested if the discrepancy cannot be resolved, if the quantity is not sufficient for a repeat, or if there is any question of a mix-up.

4. Some possible explanations for the discrepancy are
    a. Reagent strips are outdated or defective.
    b. Patient is taking large doses of vitamin C (ascorbic acid), which decreases the sensitivity of the reagent strip reaction.
    c. The structures (cells) identified as RBCs are *not* RBCs.
    d. Patient has a urinary tract infection, and nitrite (>10 mg/dL) decreases the sensitivity of the reagent strip reaction and may cause false-negatives.
    e. The specimen was not mixed adequately before dipping the reagent strip.
    f. Patient is on captopril (an antihypertensive), which has been associated with false-negatives.

5. Five possibilities for the structure identified as RBCs are WBCs, yeast, calcium oxalate crystals, oil, or air bubbles.

6. Strategies to differentiate WBCs, yeast, calcium oxalate crystals, or oil or air bubbles from RBCs follow:
    a. Add 1% acetic acid, and repeat the microscopic. RBCs will lyse, but WBCs, yeast, and oil droplets will *not* lyse; in fact, the nuclei of WBCs will be accentuated, making them easier to identify.
    b. Add Sternheimer-Malbin (S-M) or toluidine stain to accentuate the nucleus of WBCs. S-M stains RBCs, but it will not stain yeast or calcium oxalate.
    c. Scan the slide for budding yeast, which is their method of reproduction. Yeast are usually smaller and rounder than RBCs and are more variable in size.
    d. Oil or air bubbles are variable in size, uniform in appearance, and highly refractile.
    e. Examine the sediment under polarized light. Rare ovoid forms of calcium oxalate, which resemble RBCs, will polarize light; RBCs and yeast will not.

7. To rule out the explanations in question 4:
    a. Verify expiration date of the reagent strips, and run positive and negative controls.
    b. Check the urine for ascorbic acid using a reagent strip and/or review the patient's clinical history. (Is the patient taking high doses of vitamin C?)
    c. Nitrite reaction is negative.
    d. Retest on a well-mixed specimen.
    e. Call the floor to check the medical history for medications the patient is receiving.

References

Acute Glomerulonephritis. (1997). [On-line] Available: hhtp://outlinemed.com/demo/nephrol/ [1999, February 2].

American Association of Blood Banks. (1999). *Technical Manual.* 13th ed. Bethesda, Md.: AABB.

Anderson, Shauna C. & Cockayne, Susan. (1993). *Clinical Chemistry: Concepts and Applications.* Philadelphia: W. B. Saunders.

Aster, J. & Kumar, V. (1999). White cells, lymph nodes, spleen and thymus. In Cotran, R. S., Kumar, V., & Collins, T. (Eds.), *Robbins Pathologic Basis of Disease.* 6th ed. Philadelphia: W. B. Saunders.

Auerbach, A. D., & Alter, B. P. (1989). Prenatal and postnatal diagnosis of aplastic anemia. In Alter, B. P. (Ed.), *Perinatal Hematology.* London: Churchill Livingstone.

Blaney, Kathy D. & Howard, Paula R. (2000). *Basic and Applied Concepts of Immunohematology.* St. Louis: Mosby.

Bishop, Michael L., Duben-Engelkirk, Janet L., & Fody, Edward P. (2000). *Clinical Chemistry: Principles, Procedures Correlations.* 4th ed. Philadelphia: J. B. Lippincott.

Bradford, C. (2000). Cytochemistry. In Rodak, B. F. (Ed.), *Hematology: Clinical Principles and Applications.* Philadelphia: W. B. Saunders.

Broome, C. V. (1993). Listeriosis: Can we prevent it? *ASM News* 59:444–446.

Brunzel, Nancy A. (1994). *Fundamentals of Urine and Body Fluid Analysis.* Phildelphia: W. B. Saunders.

Bullock, B. L. (1996). Shock. In Bullock, B. L. (Ed.), *Pathophysiology: Adaptations and Alternations in Function.* 4th ed. Philadelphia: J. B. Lippincott.

Burtis, Carl A. & Ashwood, Edward R. (1999). *Tietz Textbook of Clinical Chemistry.* 3rd ed. Philadelphia: W. B. Saunders.

Burtis, Carl, A. & Ashwood, Edward R. (Eds.). (2001). *Tietz Fundamentals of Clinical Chemistry.* 5th ed. Philadelphia: W. B. Saunders.

Centers for Disease Control. (1999). *Epstein-Barr Virus and Infectious Mononucleosis.* [On-line] Available: http://www.cdc.gov/nciod/diseases/ebv.htm [2000, August 9].

Centers for Disease Control. (1993). *1993 Revised Classification System for HIV Infection and Expanded Surveillance Case Definition for AIDS Among Adolescents and Adults.* [On-line] Available: http://www.cdc.gov/mmwr/preview/mmwrhtml/00018871.htm [2000, November 22].

Centers for Disease Control. (1999). *Syphilis Elimination: History in the Making.* [On-line] Available: http://www.cdc.gov.nchstp/dstd/Fact_Sheets/Syphilis_Facts.htm [2000, August 11].

Clare, N. & Hansen, K. (1996). Chromosome analysis of hematopoietic disorders. In McKenzie, S. B. (Ed.), *Textbook of Hematology.* 2nd ed. Baltimore: Williams & Wilkins.

Clark, K. & Hippel, C. (2000). Routine testing in hematology. In Rodak, B. *Hematology: Clinical Principles and Applications.* 2nd ed. Philadelphia: W. B. Saunders.

Clerc, J. M. (1995). Coagulation disorders. In Rodak B. F. (Ed.), *Diagnostic Hematology.* Philadelphia: W. B. Saunders.

Damjanov, Ivan. (1996). *Pathology for the Health-Related Professions.* Philadelphia: W. B. Saunders.

Davis, Brenta G., Bishop, Michael L. & Mass, Diana (Eds.). (1989). *Clinical Laboratory Science: Strategies for Practice.* Philadelphia: J. B. Lippincott.

Dhawan, Rajiv, Jyothinagaran, Madhu G. & Shwartz, Allan B. (1999). *Pathogenesis and Management of Rhabdomyolysis.* [On-line] Available: www.auhs.edu/continuing/cme/medicine/pathogen/introduc.htm [1999, March 3].

Doig, K. (2000). Disorders of iron metabolism. In Rodak, B. F. (Ed.), *Hematology: Clinical Principles and Applications.* Philadelphia: W. B. Saunders.

Fritsma, G. (2000). Evaluation of hemostatis. In Rodak, B. F. (Ed.), *Hematology: Clinical Principles and Applications,* 2nd ed. Philadelphia: W. B. Saunders.

Fritsma G. (2000a). Evaluation of hemostasis. In Rodak B. F. (Ed.), *Hematology: Clinical Principles and Applications.* Philadelphia: W. B. Saunders.

Fritsma, G. (2000b). Hemorrhagic coagulation disorders. In Rodak B. F. (Ed.), *Hematology: Clinical Principles and Applications.* Philadelphia: W. B. Saunders.

Fritsma G. (2000c). Normal hemostasis and coagulation. In Rodak B. F. (Ed.), *Hematology: Clinical Principles and Applications.* Philadelphia: W. B. Saunders.

Fritsma, G. (2000c). Thrombotic risk testing. In Rodak, B. F. (Ed.), *Hematology: Clinical Principles and Applications.* Philadelphia: W. B. Saunders.

Graber, Mark A. & Martinez-Bianchi, Viviana. (1999). *Genitourinary and Renal Disease: Urinary Tract Infections: Females.* [On-line] Available: http://www.vh.org/Providers/ClinRef/FPHandbook/Chapter11/01-11.html [1999, March 10].

Gulley, M. L. (1996). Molecular genetics of hematologic diseases. In McKenzie, S. B. (Ed.), *Textbook of Hematology.* 2nd ed. Baltimore: Williams & Wilkins.

Handin, R. I., Lux, S. E., & Stossel, T. P. (Eds.). (1995). *Blood: Principles and Practice of Hematology.* Philadelphia: J. B. Lippincott.

Harmening, Denise M. (Ed.). (1999). *Modern Blood Banking and Transfusion Practices.* 4th ed. Philadelphia: F. A. Davis.

Harmening, Denise M. (Ed.). (1997). *Clinical Hematology and Fundamentals of Hemostasis.* 3rd ed. Philadelphia: F. A. Davis.

Healthanswers. (1999). *Pyelonephritis.* [On-line]. Available: http://www.health answers.com/database/ami/converted/000522.html [1999, February 2].

HealthAnswers. (1999). [On-line] Available: www.healthanswers.com/ Cente...w.asp?id=heart&filename=000158.htm [2000, February 24].

Hepnet. (1999). *Initial Interferon Therapy Cost-Effective for Chronic Hepatitis C Patients.* [On-line] Available: hepnet.com/hepc/news122398.html [1999, February 2].

Jaffe, Allan. (1998). *Ruling Out Myocardial Infarction with Serologic Markers.* [On-line] Available: www.medscape.com/medscape/CNO/1998/ACC/04.01 /acc0708.jaff/acc0708.jaff.html

John, K. (2000). Immunocytochemistry. In Rodak, B. F. (Ed.), *Hematology: Clinical Principles and Applications.* Philadelphia: W. B. Saunders.

Johnson, M. A., Rohlfs, E. M. & Silverman, L. M. (1999). Proteins. In Burtis, C. A. & Ashwood, E. R. (Eds.), *Tietz Textbook of Clinical Chemistry.* Philadelphia: W. B. Saunders.

Kaplan, Lawrence A., & Pesce, Amadeo J. (1996). *Clinical Chemistry: Theory, Analysis, Correlation.* 3rd ed. St. Louis: Mosby.

Kleinschmidt, Paul. (2000). *Chronic Obstructive Pulmonary Disease and Emphysema.* [On-line] Available: www.emedicine.com/emerg/topic99.htm [2000, September 5].

Koneman, Elmer W., et al. (1997). *Color Atlas and Textbook of Diagnostic Microbiology.* 5th ed. Philadelphia: J. B. Lippincott.

Kotylo, P. (2000). Lymphoproliferative disorders. In Rodak, B. F. (Ed.), *Hematology: Clinical Principles and Applications.* 3rd ed. Philadelphia: W. B. Saunders.

Kuritzkes, Daniel R. (2000). *HIV Pathogenesis and Viral Markers.* [On-line] Available: www.Medscape.com/Medscape/HIV/ClinicalMgmt/CM.v02/pnt-CM.v02.html (2000, October 27).

Larson, L. (1996a). Disorders of secondary hemostasis. In MacKenzie S. B. (Ed.), *Textbook of Hematology.* 2nd ed. Baltimore: Williams & Wilkins.

Larson, L. (1996b). Laboratory methods in coagulation. In MacKenzie S. B. (Ed.), *Textbook of Hematology.* 2nd ed. Baltimore: Williams & Wilkins.

Leclair, S. (2000). Leukopoiesis. In Rodak, B. F. (Ed.), *Hematology: Clinical Principles and Applications.* Philadelphia: W. B. Saunders.

Leclair, S. (2000). Qualitative leukocyte disorders. In Rodak, B. F. (Ed.), *Hematology: Clinical Principles and Applications.* Philadelphia: W. B. Saunders.

Leclair, S. (2000). Quantitative leukocyte disorders. In Rodak, B. F. (Ed.), *Hematology: Clinical Principles and Applications.* Philadelphia: W. B. Saunders.

Life Extension Foundation. (1999). [On-line] Available: www.lef.org/protocols/ prtcl-037.shtml [2000, February 25].

Lind, S. E. (1995). The hemostatic system. In Handin, R. I., Lux, S. E. & Stossel, T. P. (Eds.), *Blood: Principles and Practice of Hematology.* Philadelphia: J. B. Lippincott.

Lotspeich-Steininger, C. A., Stiene-Martin, E. A. & Koepke, J. A. (1992). *Clinical Hematology: Principles, Procedures, and Correlations*. Philadelphia: J. B. Lippincott.

Love, Jonathan. (2000). *Open for Discussion: Acute Pancreatitis*. [On-line] Available: www.cag-acg.org/sponsors/janssen/open_for_discussion/case25/case25.html.

Mahon, Connie R. & Manuselis, George. (1995). *Textbook of Diagnostic Microbiology*. Philadelphia: W. B. Saunders.

Mandell, Gerald L., et al. (2000). *Mandell, Douglas, and Bennett's Principles and Practice of Infectious Diseases*. 5th ed., vols 1 & 2. Philadelphia: Churchill Livingstone.

McBride, Landy J. (1998). *Textbook of Urinalysis and Body Fluids*. Philadelphia: J. B. Lippincott.

McKenzie, S. B. (1996). Nonmalignant lymphocyte disorders. In McKenzie, S. B. (Ed.), *Textbook of Hematology*. 2nd ed. Baltimore: Williams & Wilkins.

McKenzie, S. B. (1996a). The erythrocyte. In *Textbook of Hematology*. 2nd ed. Baltimore: Williams & Wilkins.

McKenzie, S. B. (1996b). Myeloproliferative disorders. In *Textbook of Hematology*. 2nd ed. Baltimore: Williams & Wilkins.

McKenzie, S. B. (1996c). Anemia of defective heme synthesis. *Textbook of Hematology*. 2nd ed. Baltimore: Williams & Wilkins.

McKenzie, S. B. (1996d). Nonmalignant granulocyte and monocyte disorders. *Textbook of Hematology*. 2nd ed. Baltimore: Williams & Wilkins.

Miller, K. (2000). Molecular diagnostics. In Rodak, B. F. (Ed.), *Hematology: Clinical Principles and Applications*. Philadelphia: W. B. Saunders.

Miller, K. (2000). Molecular diagnostics. In Rodak, B. F. (Ed.), *Hematology: Clinical Principles and Applications*. Philadelphia: W. B. Saunders.National Academy of Clinical Biochemistry. (1998). *Use of Cardiac Markers in Coronary Artery Disease*. [On-line] Available: www.nacb.org/nacb_SOLP_ [1998, October 6].

Murray, Patrick R., et al. (1995). *Manual of Clinical Microbiology*. 6th ed. Washington D.C.: ASM Press.

National Academy of Clinical Biochemistry. (1998). *Use of Cardiac Markers in Coronary Artery Disease*. [On-line] Available: www.nacb.org/nacb_SOLP_ [1998, October 6].

National Cholesterol Education Program (NCEP). (1993). *Second Report of the Expert Panel on Detection, Evaluation, and Treatment of High Cholesterol in Adults (Adult Treatment Panel II)*. [On-line] Available: www.nhlbi.nih.gov/duidelines/cholesterol/atp_sum.htm (2000, November 6).

National Institute of Arthritis and Musculoskeletal Diseases. (1999). *Handout on Health—Rheumatoid Arthritis*. [On-line] Available: http://pharminfor.com/disease/ra/ra_handout.html [2000, August 28].

Niederu, Claus, Lange, Stefan, Heintges, Tobias, et al. (1999). *Prognosis of Chronic Hepatitis C: Results of a Large, Prospective Cohort Study*. [On-line] Available: www.hepatology.org./cgi.content/full/ [1999, February 3].

Pittman, Joel R. & Bross, Michael H. (1999). *Diagnosis and Management of Gout.* [On-line] Available: www.aafp.org/afp/990401ap/1799.html [2000, September 5].

Quinley, Eva D. (1998). *Immunohematology: Principles and Practice.* 2nd ed. Philadelphia: J. B. Lippincott.

Ringsrud, Karen Munson & Jorgenson Linne, Jean. (1995). *Urinalysis and Body Fluids: A Color Text and Atlas.* St. Louis: Mosby.

RxMed. (1999). *Nephrotic Syndrome.* [On-line] Available: http://www.rxmed.com/illnesses/nephrotic_syndrome.html [1999, February 8].

Santen, Sally. (2000). *Cholecystitis and Biliary Colic.* [On-line] Available: www.emedicine.com/emerg/topic98.htm (2000, September 5).

Sheehan, Catherine. (1997). *Clinical Immunology: Principles and Laboratory Diagnosis.* Philadelphia: J. B. Lippincott.

Stevens, Christine Dorresteyn. (1996). *Clinical Immunology and Serology: A Laboratory Perspective.* Philadelphia: F. A. Davis.

Strasinger, Susan King. (1994). *Urinalysis and Body Fluids.* Philadelphia: F. A. Davis.

Turgeon, Mary Louis. (1996). *Immunology and Serology in Laboratory Medicine.* St. Louis: Mosby.

Vance, G. (2000). Cytogenetics. In Rodak, B. F. (Ed.), *Hematology: Clinical Principles and Applications.* Philadelphia: W. B. Saunders.

WebMD. (1999). *Systemic Lupus Erythematosus.* [On-line] Available: http://webmed.lycos.com/content/dmk/dmk_article_4056 (2000, October 3).

Wiersinga, W. M., & DeGroot, Leslie J. (1999). "Chapter 9. Adult Hypothyroidism." [On-line] Available: www.thyroidmanager.og/Chapter9/9-text.htm (2000, July 5).